The Ultimate Instant Pot®
Cookbook for Two

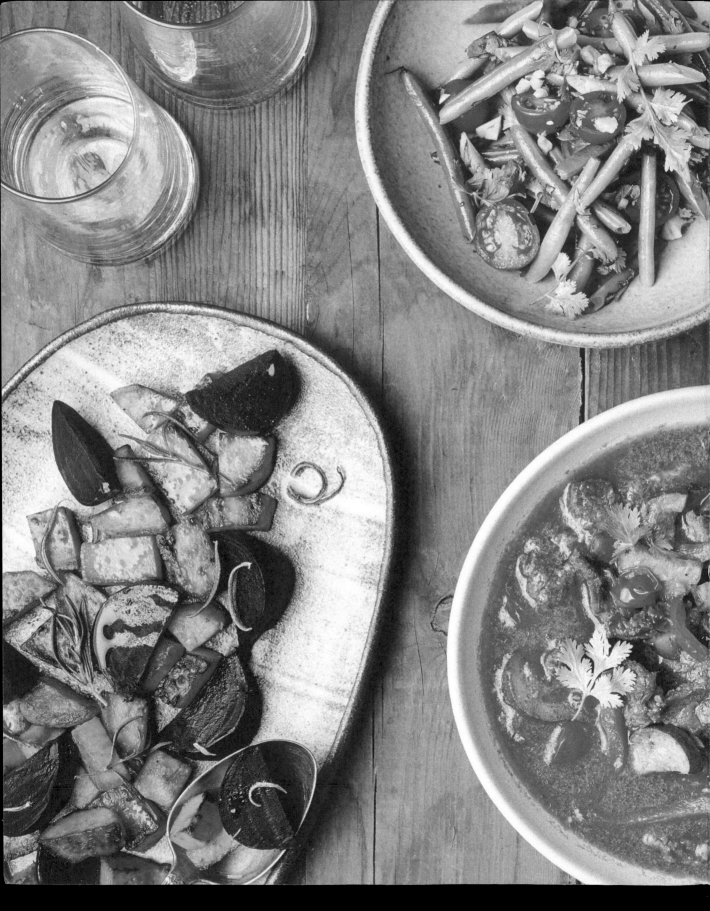

The ULTIMATE Instant Pot® COOKBOOK *for two*

Perfectly Portioned Recipes for 3-Quart and 6-Quart Models

JANET A. ZIMMERMAN
Author of *Instant Pot® Obsession*

Photography by Marija Vidal

ROCKRIDGE PRESS

Interior and Cover Designer: Jamison Spittler
Photo Art Director / Art Manager: Sue Smith
Editor: Stacy Wagner-Kinnear
Production Editor: Erum Khan
Photography by Marija Vidal, © 2018, food styling by Cregg Green

ISBN: Print 978-1-64152-388-2 | eBook 978-1-64152-389-9

To my late parents,
Rene and Larry Zimmerman,
who, in very different ways,
taught me about food and cooking.

And to Dave,
who kept everything going while
I was writing the book.

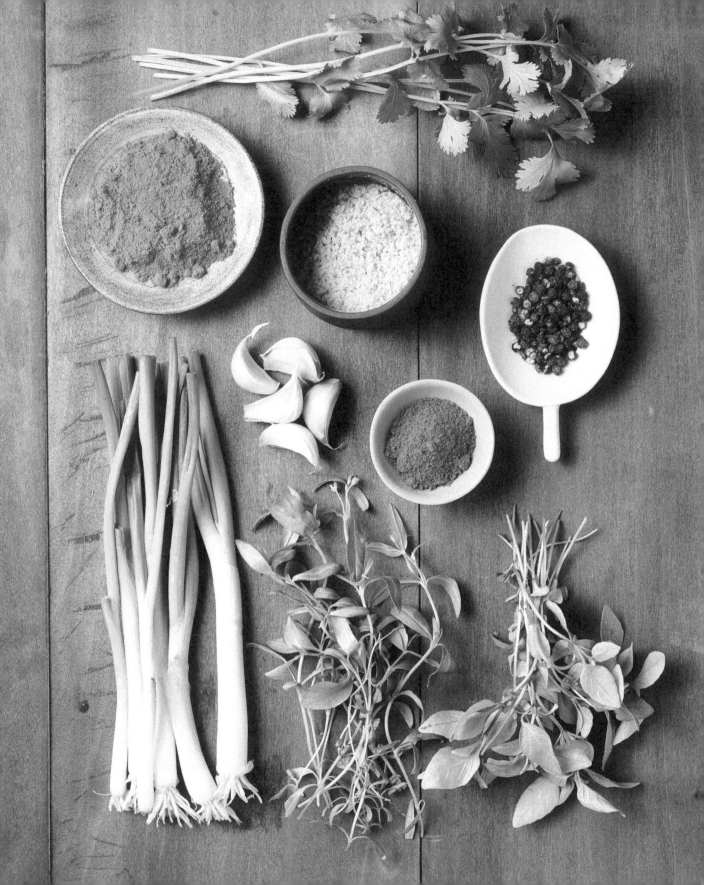

contents

Introduction . . . ix

1

Cooking for Two Made Easy . . . 1

2

Breakfast . . . 21

3

Vegetables and Sides . . . 37

4

Beans and Grains . . . 55

5

Meatless Mains . . . 73

6

Seafood and Poultry . . . 89

7

Beef and Pork . . . 121

8

Desserts . . . 143

9

Kitchen Staples . . . 157

Instant Pot® Pressure Cooking Time Charts . . . 169

Measurement Conversions . . . 175

Recipe Index . . . 176

Index . . . 178

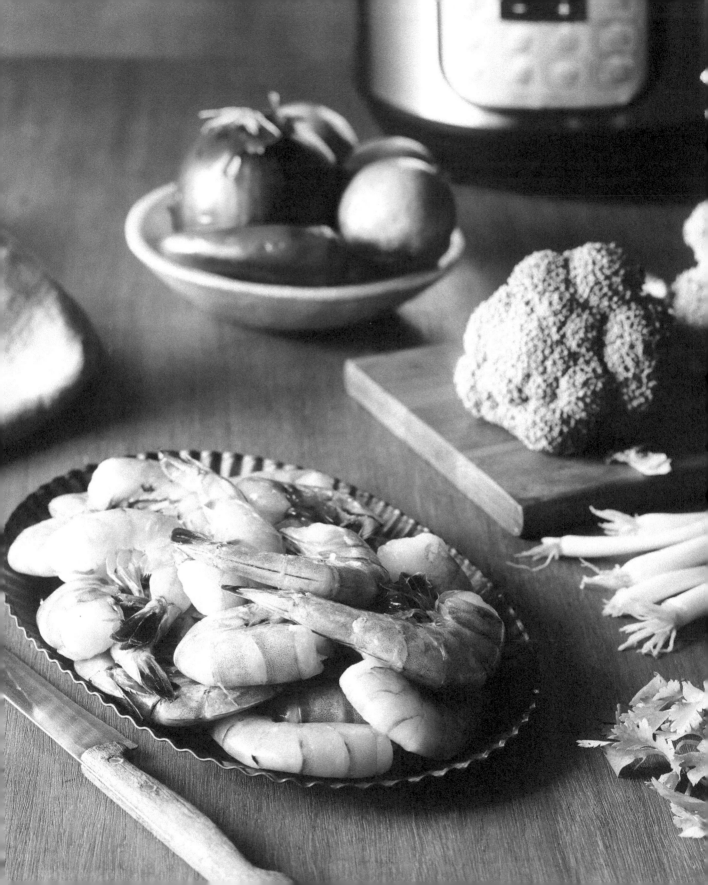

introduction

This book is near and dear to my heart. I cook for two nearly every night, and have for most of my adult life. I've also spent much of my professional cooking career developing recipes for two.

One cooking appliance I've long relied on when developing recipes for myself and others is the pressure cooker. I wrote *The Healthy Pressure Cooker Cookbook* in 2015 to make pressure cooking with a stove-top or electric pressure cooker easy for everybody. It published just as buzz about the Instant Pot® was heating up. Like so many other cooks, I've mostly shelved my trusty stove-top pressure cookers. Walk through my kitchen and you'll find not one, not two, but three different Instant Pot® models. Needless to say, it was a natural and enjoyable process to expand my pressure cooking expertise with the Instant Pot®. My second pressure cooking cookbook, *Instant Pot® Obsession*, published in early 2017, and it's been very well received.

Somewhere along the way, though, pressure cookers have become known for big batches of food—pots of chili or stew for a crowd, pounds of meat cooked in minutes, or huge batches of beans or pasta. Many people seem unsure about using the Instant Pot® for "just two." It doesn't help that there are so few reliable pressure cooker recipes out there for two people. Let's face it, these days so-called Instant Pot® experts are thick on the ground. Some of their recipes work; some, well, not so much. And it's even worse for small-batch recipes. The few that can be found online seem destined for failure, and the cookbook offerings for two have been sketchy at best.

That's where this cookbook comes in. Not only do I include a wide variety of great recipes for two, I also offer tips that'll help you shop for two, plan your meals, and deal with recipes that unavoidably make some leftovers. Once you get started, I trust you'll agree that your Instant Pot®—together with this book—will make cooking for two as quick, easy, and enjoyable as I know it can be.

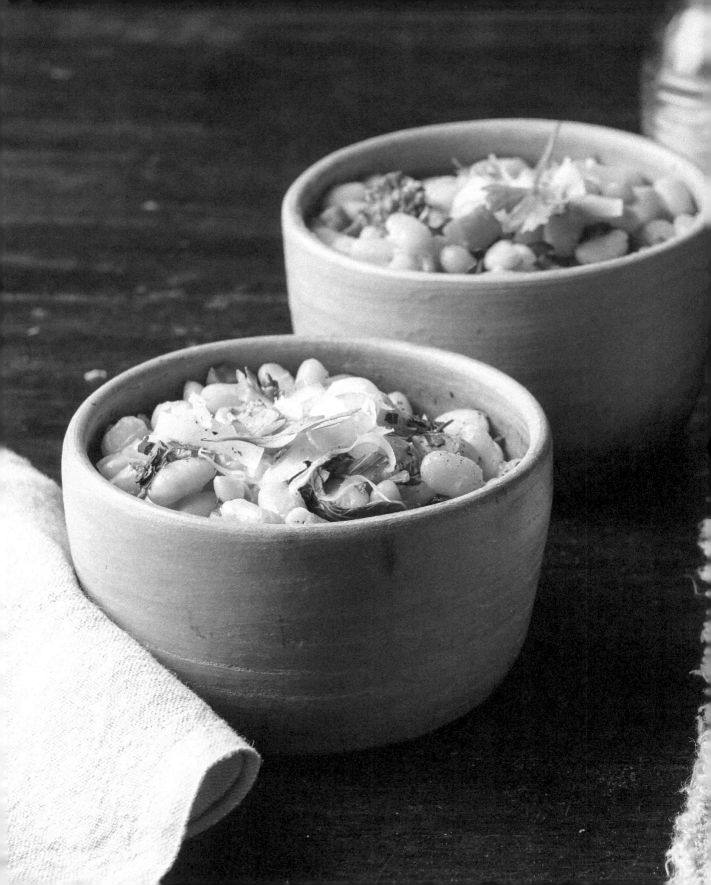

chapter 1
Cooking for Two Made Easy

For many people, especially couples, dinner is the best time to spend time together, enjoying a meal while you catch up on the day. But whether you're cooking for a spouse, partner, child, or roommate, it can be daunting to cook dinner every night. You want to make sure your meals are nutritious and satisfying, but you're probably pressed for time. Because it's just two of you, it can be tempting to let cooking slide and order takeout or fast food instead. The time the Instant Pot® gives back to people, not to mention the hands-off convenience, is a huge part of why it's been such a revelation for home cooks everywhere.

White Bean Stew with Broccoli Rabe, page 56

My "For Two" Philosophy

I'll let you in on a secret. Cooking for two is much easier than cooking for a crowd, or even a small family—especially with an Instant Pot®. The more people you cook for, the more variables you have to contend with—who had a late snack, who skipped lunch, or who's feeling sick—not to mention all the food likes and dislikes. But with two, once you know your appetites, it's a breeze to cook exactly the right amount of food. No leftovers, unless you want them.

The recipes in this book may yield some leftovers; that's because I write them for "average" appetites. I don't want you to go hungry, so I tend to err on the side of too much rather than too little. As you cook through the book, you can make notes on the amounts you prefer and use those as guidelines for future meals. In a few cases, it's difficult to cook just two servings—with some desserts, for example. In those cases, the leftovers will keep for a couple of days, or can be used in further meals. (And who doesn't like having extra dessert?)

At first glance, it might seem that a pressure cooker is made for larger meals—big pots of stew, pulled pork for a crowd, racks of ribs. But it's just as great for making small batches. Even better, in some ways. The less food you have in your Instant Pot®, the faster it will come to pressure. Without a pot full of food, you can get by with less liquid, which means your stews won't be watery and your sauces won't need thickening. If you've never used your Instant Pot® to cook for two, you'll be amazed at what it can do.

Instant Pot® 101

If you already own an Instant Pot® (or maybe more than one), you know how they work and what they can do. If you're new to the Instant Pot® world, here's a quick rundown of their features and capabilities.

The Instant Pot® is an electric multicooker, which means it has several cooking programs. It can function as a pressure cooker (the most popular function), rice cooker, slow cooker, and yogurt maker. There are preprogrammed settings for various foods, which start with the touch of one button. Or you can customize the cooking process with the Pressure Cook setting (or Manual, if you own an older model). Either way, the Instant Pot® is a game changer for today's cooks.

Here are just a few of its advantages:

Speed. Pressure cooking can cut traditional cooking times by half or even more. Think pot roast in 60 minutes, unsoaked dry beans in 45 minutes, or a complete pasta dinner in 25 minutes.

Hands-off cooking. No more standing in front of the stove, adjusting the heat, and stirring constantly. With the Instant Pot®, even a labor-intensive dish like risotto can cook almost entirely unattended.

Energy savings. With so many one-pot possibilities, you won't need multiple burners and the oven to get dinner on the table. This saves energy and helps keep your kitchen cool on the hottest summer days.

Healthier meal options. The speed and the convenience of the Instant Pot® mean there's no need to order takeout or rely on prepackaged frozen dinners. You can cook healthier meals from scratch in about the same amount of time, all while controlling the ingredients you use.

Safety. The Instant Pot® has multiple safety features. It automatically regulates the temperature and pressure with no oversight required. You can set it, walk away, and know there's nothing to worry about.

Terms to Know

As you become familiar with your Instant Pot®, there may be a few new terms.

Pressure release valve: The valve on the lid that controls the release of steam and pressure. In some models, it toggles between Sealing and Venting (in these recipes, it should always be set to Sealing). In the Ultra models, it's set to Sealing by default.

Sealing ring: The silicone ring that fits around the lid's underside that seals the pot so pressure can build. It's crucial for this to be free of nicks or tears and placed correctly before the lid goes on.

Seal: When the pot comes to pressure, the lid will be sealed on the pot. Never try to remove a sealed lid.

Pot-in-pot cooking: Cooking method in which ingredients are placed in a bowl or other cooking dish, which is then placed on a trivet above water for steaming.

High pressure: The high pressure setting is between 10.2 and 11.6 PSI (which produces cooking temperatures between 240°F and 245°F).

Low pressure: Available on all models except the Lux, low pressure is between 6 and 7 PSI (which produces a cooking temperature of 230°F).

Sauté: A setting to brown meats or vegetables or simmer sauces that can be set to low, medium, or high heat.

Steam: The Steam setting heats faster and more constantly than Pressure Cook or Manual settings, so the pot will come to pressure faster.

Pressure cook/manual: Depending on the model, there is either a Pressure Cook or Manual setting, used for customized cooking times.

Natural release: After cooking, this allows the pressure inside the pot come down on its own, which can take 10 to 30 minutes depending on the contents.

Quick release: After cooking, the pressure can be released immediately by flipping the valve to Vent (or pressing the Quick Release button on the Ultra model).

Venting: The release valve setting that allows steam to escape. It's used to release pressure after cooking, and in slow cooking and yogurt making.

Keep warm: This default setting (which can be disabled) keeps food warm after cooking. In some models, the temperature is adjustable.

Cooking the Instant Pot® Way

Once you get the hang of using the Instant Pot®, you'll be cooking like a pro in no time. Here's a rundown of some of the usual prep and cooking steps, in the order in which you're likely to complete them.

1. **Precook ingredients.** With some recipes, you'll need to precook. What's wonderful is that you can do it all in the Instant Pot®; there's no need for a skillet. First, you'll remove the lid and set it aside or conveniently hinge it on one of the side handles of the cooker base of the Instant Pot® (yes, those handles can double as storage if you place the lid

vertically into one of them). Then you'll brown meat or sauté vegetables using the Sauté function. If there are any bits of food stuck to the pot, you'll add a bit of liquid and scrape the pot to unstick them.

2. **Add liquid and/or the remaining ingredients.** To pressure steam foods like eggs, vegetables, or desserts, first you'll add water and the trivet or steaming basket. The food will go in a bowl or basket above the water. To pressure cook foods directly, such as stews, pasta, and meat dishes, you'll put the ingredients right into the inner cooking pot, along with enough liquid to allow the pot to come to pressure.

3. **Lock the lid into place.** Once the lid is locked, you'll set the release valve to Sealing so that the pot can come to pressure.

4. **Select the cooking function, adjust the pressure, and input the cooking time.** Regardless of which cooking function you select, the pot will display a default time. You can adjust this using the [+] or [-] buttons to increase or decrease time. Depending on the model, you may or may not have to press a start button. The Ultra has one; other models do not. If there is no start button, a few seconds after you select set the cooking time the display screen will display ON, which lets you know the pot is working to build pressure.

5. **Release pressure.** Once the cooking time finishes, you'll either let the pressure release naturally (meaning the pot cools down on its own) or you'll be instructed to do what's called a quick release by flipping the pressure release valve to Venting. In some instances, you'll let the pressure release naturally for a specified time and then flip the valve to Venting to quickly release the remaining steam.

6. **Finish the dish.** Some recipes will need finishing to bring the dish together. In this book, finishing instructions will have you thickening sauces, adding quick cooking ingredients, or adjusting the seasoning.

PRESSURE
RELEASE VALVE

FLOAT VALVE

LID

Instant Pot® DUO Mini

Soup
Broth

Rice

Meat
Stew

Low Pressure High

Less Normal More

COOKER BASE

Steam

Bean
Chili

− +

Slow
Cook

Pressure
Level

Keep
Warm

Yogurt

Saute

Delay
Start

Cancel

Pressure
Cook

TRIVET

www.InstantPot.com

RAMEKINS

MEASURING CUP

STEAMER BASKET

SEALING RING

INNER COOKING POT

BAKING DISH

SPRINGFORM PAN

Which Model Is Right for Two?

Instant Pot® models have come a long way from the early days. At first there was only a 5- or 6-quart Lux model. Now there are four sizes, from the 3-quart Mini to the 8-quart models. With so many choices, what's the best pot for two?

No matter the size of your Instant Pot®, you can successfully cook for two. All the recipes in this book were tested in either the 3-quart or 6-quart Instant Pot® (Ultra and Duo). The 8-quart pot is just a bit too big for some of these recipes. If you have the older Lux 5-quart model, which only cooks on high pressure, it will work as well, although there are a few recipes using low pressure that require some modifications, which I provide.

I use the 6-quart Ultra model the most. With my Ultra, I don't have to remember to set the valve to Sealing, it's easier to quick release the pressure, and the screen includes a graphic readout of the cooking progress. (The Ultra can also calculate timing alterations for high altitudes.) But you can feel confident cooking these recipes with any 3-, 5-, or 6-quart model you have.

The Skinny on the Mini

When Instant Pot® introduced the 3-quart Mini in 2017, it seemed tailor-made for cooks wanting to prepare smaller recipes, as well as those with kitchen space limitations. Is it the perfect match for two?

Models: Like the 6-quart, the Mini is available in Lux, Duo, Duo Plus, and Ultra models.

Recipe yields: The Mini is ideal for cooking small batches or rice or other grains, and it can be useful for side dishes for two. Some main dish recipes for two will work fine; but you may find that for entrées like pasta, you'll be at the maximum fill line before you know it.

Speed: I know what you're thinking: It's smaller, so it must heat up more quickly. But that's not the case. The Mini draws less power (700 watts compared with 1,000 for the 6-quart), and the same volume of liquid ingredients will be deeper, both of which cause it to heat more slowly. In my tests, 2 cups of liquid took 1 to 2 minutes longer to come to pressure in the Mini than in the 6-quart. This is not a deal-breaker; but you may have to adjust some recipes with short cooking times (which I've done for you in these recipes).

Space: If your kitchen is tiny or space is at a premium, the Mini might be a better option. It's about 2 inches smaller in diameter and 2 inches shorter (with lid) than the 6-quart.

Supporting Equipment

Experienced Instant Pot® users know that buying the pot is just the beginning. It's easy to go overboard buying accessories, but my list of essential equipment is short.

Baking dish. My go-to is a ceramic, straight-sided, 1-quart soufflé dish. Any metal, oven-safe glass, or ceramic dish or bowl will work as long as it holds at least 3 cups. The diameter should be up to 7 inches for the 6-quart and 6 inches or less for the 3-quart.

Individual ramekins, custard cups, or small jars. Great for some breakfast and dessert recipes, they should hold 6 to 8 ounces with a diameter of about 4 inches for the 6-quart or 3 inches for the 3-quart. Silicone cups work as long as they are the right size and hold their shape. Larger ramekins (1½ cups) are also useful.

Springform pan. A 7-inch pan fits the 6-quart pot; for the 3-quart, it should be 6 inches or smaller. Alternatively, use a cake pan with a removable bottom. Mini springform pans (4 inches) can also be useful.

Steamer basket. I like the silicone models with locking handles. For these recipes, you don't need a big, deep basket; the shallow ones work fine.

Trivets. All Instant Pot® models come with a trivet, but it might be worth buying one or two more. The trivets in the newer models have handles, but for older models, a trivet with handles is a good investment. There is even a silicone model. I also find it handy to have a tall trivet when cooking one food in a bowl over food in the bottom. It should be about 3 inches high.

Other useful tools include an immersion blender, food scale (for pasta and meat), sturdy tongs, fat separator, and silicone finger mitts for removing the inner pot or securing it while you stir ingredients.

Planning Meals for Two

When you're cooking for two, menu planning involves more than just figuring out what your meals will be for the week and then buying the ingredients. Because you'll use smaller amounts of some ingredients, you'll want to develop a strategy for using up the rest before they go bad. This can be especially important with produce and some proteins. If you buy a whole head of cabbage, for instance, you'll need a plan to use it all within about two weeks.

The recipes in this book may only use half a can of tomatoes or beans, or half a fennel bulb, or part of a bag of spinach. In those cases, I will point you to another recipe that uses the rest, or at least provide some ideas for using up the remainder.

Consider dividing ingredients that can be frozen, and labeling and dating them. I use a whiteboard on the freezer to keep track of what's in there, but you don't have to be that obsessive. As you do your weekly planning, check your supplies and choose recipes that use up some of the older ingredients rather than buy new ones.

How Much for Two?

When cooking for two, it's important to know how much food to prepare, which means knowing how much you will actually eat. Here are some general guidelines I use in my recipes, which yield two generous servings. To cook the right portions for you and your dining partner, pay attention to how much you both eat, take notes, and then weigh or measure your food before cooking.

Grains and Pasta

For most grains, plan for ⅓ to ½ cup of raw grains for two average-to-generous servings (grains expand three to four times as they cook). It can be tricky to pressure cook the smaller amount unless you cook pot-in-pot, so most of these recipes call for at least a ½ cup. For dried pasta, 4 ounces will yield two average servings—6 ounces is generous and 8 ounces is huge. With all the shapes and sizes of pasta, weighing is the best way to get an accurate amount.

Beans

The amount of beans for two servings varies depending on whether they constitute a side dish or an entrée, as well as what else is in the dish. Plan on 4 ounces for two servings of a side dish or soups with other ingredients, and 6 to 8 ounces for two main dish servings. See page 162 (Basic Beans) for more information on bean serving sizes.

Proteins

Protein serving sizes vary depending on how rich the protein source is, and whether or not it contains bones or lots of fat or connective tissue, which will be discarded. For two servings, you'll probably want between 8 and 12 ounces of boneless lean meat, fish, or tofu. For heartier meats that contain bones or connective tissue, like pork shoulder or beef ribs, you'll need 1½ to 2 pounds.

Vegetables

Vegetable serving sizes depend on several factors: the type of vegetable, whether it's served raw or cooked, and what else you're eating with it. Leafy vegetables lose much of their mass when cooked; a serving of cooked spinach might be twice as much (by weight) as a serving of raw spinach. In general, count on 2 cups of raw leafy greens or about 1 cup of cooked vegetables for two servings.

Go-To Ingredients

There are a few ingredients that show up in multiple recipes in this book. Here are some foods that I use regularly in my Instant Pot®, especially in recipes for two.

Chicken thighs. Whether bone-in with skin or boneless and skinless, chicken thighs are a great choice for the Instant Pot®. They're cheaper than chicken breast, tastier, and much more forgiving if slightly overcooked.

Chuck roast. Beef shoulder (also known as chuck) is a versatile choice for pressure cooking. Blade roasts are a relatively small, compact cut of shoulder. Whatever cut I buy, I usually cut it into 2-inch chunks or strips, so it cooks more quickly.

Condiments and sauces. I don't use many premade sauces, but I do use hoisin sauce, soy sauce, Asian chili-garlic sauce, and Sriracha. I use jarred salsa in some Mexican and Southwestern recipes (Frontera brand). I always have at least one hot sauce on hand, usually Tabasco or Crystal. Dijon or whole-grain mustards make appearances in these recipes. I use a variety of vinegars, extra-virgin olive oil, dry red and white wine (four-packs of small bottles are a great option), and dry sherry. Worcestershire sauce, anchovy paste, and Marmite add umami (savory) flavors, and I use liquid smoke, chipotles, and smoked paprika to lend a smoky hint to dishes that are commonly grilled.

County-style shoulder ribs. These are strips of pork shoulder, sometimes with bones, sometimes boneless. Pork shoulder is perfect for pressure cooking, and using country ribs is a great way to buy pork shoulder for two. Be careful, though—some butchers cut up pork loin and sell that as country ribs, and loin is not a great choice for pressure cooking.

Dairy products. While there are plenty of dairy-free recipes in this book, many will call for butter, heavy (whipping) cream, whole milk, sour cream, and a variety of cheeses.

Where recipes do call for dairy, I've made an effort to include suggestions for dairy-free alternatives.

Freezer. Two of my favorite freezer items are individually frozen (IQF) shell-on shrimp and tilapia or cod fillets. I also use frozen peas and frozen corn. I always have a container of orange juice concentrate—it's an easy way to add a hint of orange to desserts or salad dressing. In a pinch, it can be reconstituted and used instead of freshly squeezed orange juice.

Garlic and ginger. I use a lot of ginger, and even more garlic. I generally press or grate them as I need them, but there are options for busy cooks. The best I've found are frozen cubes (I've used the Dorot Gardens brand), but other brands are available in tubes or jars.

Pantry goods. Pantry items include canned goods like diced tomatoes, strained tomatoes, canned beans, dried beans, pasta, and rice.

Spices. In so many cases, spices make the dish, so it's important to have at least a basic selection. If you can't count on your local supermarket or international market to stock them, you can order online from companies like Penzeys or the Savory Spice House. Basics I recommend include ancho chile powder, celery seed, mustard seed, kosher salt (these recipes are developed with Diamond brand), cumin, Chinese five-spice powder, black peppercorns, and fresh nutmeg.

Essential Shopping Tips

When shopping for two, a regular grocery store can seem like a big box store—everything comes in larger sizes than you need. The following tips can help you navigate grocery stores and avoid waste when shopping.

- **Find the best-fit stores.** If possible, shop at a market near a college or university, or in a section of town populated primarily by singles and couples. Look for a market with actual meat and seafood counters, where you can buy individual steaks or fillets.

- **Get to know the staff.** Ask questions and be polite, and you'll find that they're happy to help you buy the amount of food you want. Don't see a half-pound package of ground beef? Ask the woman behind the meat counter, and she'll probably package it for you. If you ask the man stocking produce, he might be willing to cut a cabbage or a butternut squash in half for you.

GETTING REAL ABOUT LEFTOVERS

Most people think of leftovers as the rest of the batch of chili in the refrigerator, or the extra serving of mashed potatoes that no one ate. But that's only one type of leftover food: extra servings, whether planned or unplanned, of prepared food. The good news when you're cooking for two is that when you follow reliable recipes (like the ones in this book!), you can usually avoid these leftovers unless you want them.

For me, there's another category of leftover food that's much more useful—basic ingredients cooked in advance and then used later on. Here's a common example: You roast a chicken on Sunday, eat part of it, and then make chicken curry or club sandwiches later in the week. In this book, I offer suggestions for a couple of ingredients cooked all at once and then used in different meals, like steamed broccoli rabe that can be used in stews, pasta, or sandwiches.

A third type of leftover food is raw ingredients that you don't use all at once. When you're cooking for two, it's pretty much impossible to use a whole head of lettuce in one meal. Likewise, if you buy a chunk of pork shoulder (or even a smaller pork tenderloin), it might well be enough meat for two or more meals. Fortunately, if you plan a little bit ahead, these leftovers are a breeze to deal with. With meat, divide it before cooking and freeze what you're not using. With vegetables, you can usually store the unused portion for a few days, at which point you can use the rest in a new recipe.

While you won't always be able to avoid leftovers, you'll often be able to choose what form those leftovers will take.

- **Buy dry goods and spices in bulk.** If your market sells goods like nuts, grains, and spices in bulk, buy from those bins. Not only can you purchase exactly the amount you need, but you'll likely save money since bulk items are often cheaper than packaged goods.

- **Purchase prepared foods wisely.** Many supermarkets today have lots of prepared foods for sale—not only meats and cheese at the deli counter, but often cut and washed produce at the salad bar or in the produce department. It can be tempting to rely on these foods, but you may be better off skipping them. The cut produce at the salad bar, for instance, is not only much more expensive than the whole items in the produce department, but it also may not be very fresh. On the other hand, if all you need is a cup or so of cabbage and you know you'll never use the whole head, buying shredded cabbage at the salad bar could very well be your best option.

- **Don't forget the frozen foods section.** Many fruits and vegetables freeze quite well, and those packages of frozen produce will last much longer than their fresh counterparts. Bags of chopped vegetables or individually frozen raw shrimp or fish fillets can be a boon when cooking for two.

Instant Pot® Troubleshooting and Questions

I'm getting a "Burn" message. Why?

When a high temperature is detected at the bottom of the inner pot, its temperature sensor suspends heating. Early models show the message "ovHt" (overheat) and newer models show "burn." I think "overheat" is a more accurate warning, since it's not always, or even usually, burning food that causes the issue. It's likely a faulty seal or the sealing valve set to the Vent position rather than Seal position, either of which will keep the pot from coming to pressure and evaporate the liquid inside. Heating the pot empty before adding your ingredients can also cause the sensor to suspend heating, as can failing to scrape up any cooked bits of food from the sautéing process.

If you get the "burn" message, release any pressure, check the seal and valve, and check to see if there is food stuck to the bottom of the pot. Then—and this is important—let the pot cool off before starting again. The fastest way to do this is to take the inner pot out for a few minutes before resuming.

Why don't your recipes always include a cup of liquid?

There's virtually no loss of liquid in a pressure cooker, so it doesn't take much to create the steam necessary to keep the pot at pressure. Proteins and vegetables release liquid as they cook, so those recipes don't need a full cup to start. A pound of raw meat, for instance, will release over ⅓ cup of liquid as it cooks—that's why pot roasts and pulled pork always have so much liquid at the end of the cooking process. Unless cooking foods that absorb water (grains, beans, or pasta), you don't need to start with the full cup needed when steaming foods. Too much liquid not only increases the time it takes for the pot to reach pressure, it results in watery, underseasoned food.

Why do you always use the Pressure Cook or Manual setting? Why not use the other cooking programs?

While the preprogrammed settings can be handy, different models have different settings. The safest bet when I'm developing recipes is not to depend on a setting that's not universally available. I do occasionally use the Steam setting, since all models have that one. As you cook through the recipes, you should feel free to use the preprogrammed functions whenever appropriate.

Why does my pot take forever to come to pressure?

When you're waiting for that pin to come up and the countdown to start, it can seem like ages. The good news is, you'll find that the time is not long when you're cooking small batches—smaller amounts take less time to heat up. When testing these recipes, the time to pressure was always under 10 minutes—usually under 8 (a little longer for the Mini). But all kinds of things can affect the process, like the temperature of your ingredients. The one thing that still throws me is when the pressure pin pops up 1 to 2 minutes before the timing countdown starts. I always tell myself: "Patience, grasshopper." If, with the recipes in this book, your pot hasn't started counting down within 12 minutes, something's probably wrong. Check the sealing ring and the valve.

Why do some of your recipes call for 0 minutes of pressure cooking? Is that a typo?

Remember that the pot begins heating immediately when it's turned on, so cooking begins well before the pot comes to pressure. And even with a quick release, you'll get an extra minute or so of cooking as the pressure releases. In some instances, that amount of cooking is all that's needed—as in the case of fast-cooking shrimp or vegetables—so 0 minutes is the right time to use.

Let's Get Cooking

The recipes in this book are written for two. Most produce two generous portions, or two moderate portions with some leftovers (for a lunch or a light dinner). Some of the dessert recipes yield two large servings or four smaller servings.

Most recipes take less than 45 minutes to prepare, and that includes time for the pot to come to pressure, as well as release it. Even the longer recipes will take less time than using conventional methods, and they often include unattended cooking time, so you won't be tied to the kitchen the entire time.

With few exceptions, the recipes take 10 minutes or less of prep time before cooking starts, and I try to include shortcuts when they won't affect the quality of the finished recipe. Whenever it saves time to prep some ingredients while other ingredients cook, I give instructions for the prep sequence. I've also tried to use ingredients a typical pantry will include; when more exotic ingredients are called for, I provide substitutes.

Most of the recipes require the same cooking and release time whether you're using a 6-quart Instant Pot® or the Mini. When the time or instructions do vary, I include complete notes on what's different. I also include separate directions for the Lux model whenever necessary.

Each recipe includes a breakdown of the time required, including prep and finishing time, sautéing time (when appropriate), time under pressure, natural release time (if any), and the total time. The total time includes the average time it takes the pot to come to pressure, generally less than 10 minutes, and time to quick release pressure, usually about a minute. In all cases, I've rounded up. Remember that several factors can affect the cooking process, such as the temperature of liquids, size of ingredients, or altitude. With longer cooking times, this doesn't make much difference, but for recipes with short cooking times, you may need to adjust the cooking time up or down by a minute or two.

All the recipes are followed by useful tips, including (when appropriate):

* Time-saving tips

* Ways to use leftover ingredients

* Dividing the labor when working with a partner

* How to increase the yield of a recipe, including changes in times and ingredients

* Recipe modifications, if relevant, when cooking with the Mini or Lux model

* Notes on accommodating common food allergies and sensitivities whenever possible

* Suggestions for recipes that pair well together, often using an additional Instant Pot®

Cooking for two is dear to my heart, and I had fun developing these recipes. I've tried to come up with recipes for all tastes and cooking styles. I hope you enjoy making them as much as I do!

SCALING RECIPES DOWN AND UP

The recipes in this book are all written for two servings. But what if you want to double them for company or to have leftovers? What if you want to convert other recipes written for four or more servings down to two? When cooking under pressure, there are a few things to keep in mind.

Water. Regardless of scaling up or down, the one thing that will never change is the amount of water in the bottom of the pot when you're steaming food on the trivet or in a steamer basket. If you're steaming 3 ounces of green beans or 6 ounces, 4 eggs or 8 eggs, you'll use the same 1 cup of water.

Doubling. When you have a recipe for two that works, simply double everything. As long as the ingredients are cut the same, the cooking times generally won't change. The exception is when there's a very short cooking time. The extra ingredients may cause the pot to take longer to come to pressure, which can mean overcooking if the time is 5 minutes or less, such as the Minestrone (page 74) or the Spicy Sesame Noodles and Vegetables (page 85). But mostly, it's easy to remember—double the ingredients, don't change the time. If you do find the dish is overcooked, subtract 1 minute from the pressure cooking time, then test the ingredients to see if they are to your preference.

Scaling down. Scaling large recipes down is a bit trickier. In most cases, you can cut recipe ingredients in half to scale down to two servings, but there are a few things to look out for. One is liquid. With pressure cooking, you need liquid boiling to reach pressure. Depending on the other ingredients, you don't need much, but the total liquid should never be less than ¼ to ½ cup. Meats and vegetables exude water as they cook, so you can easily get by with the smaller amount. Don't halve the oil or butter when it's used to sauté or brown ingredients. You'll need enough to cover the bottom of the pot, so you won't want to cut those ingredients past that point. As with doubled recipes, the cooking time will usually remain the same, but remember that with a smaller volume in the pot, it will take less time to come to pressure. You may occasionally need to increase the cooking time to account for that.

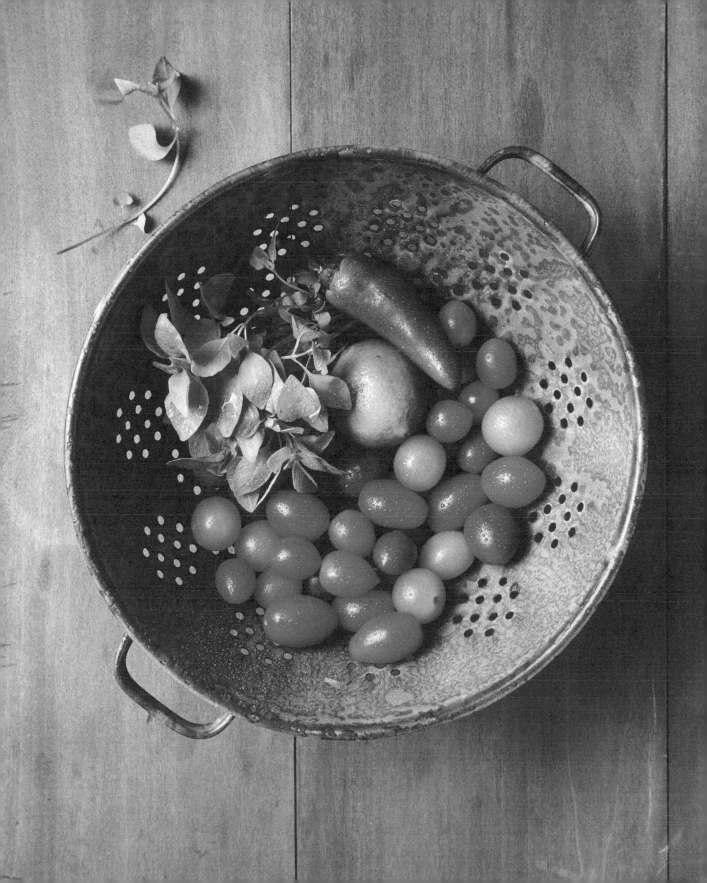

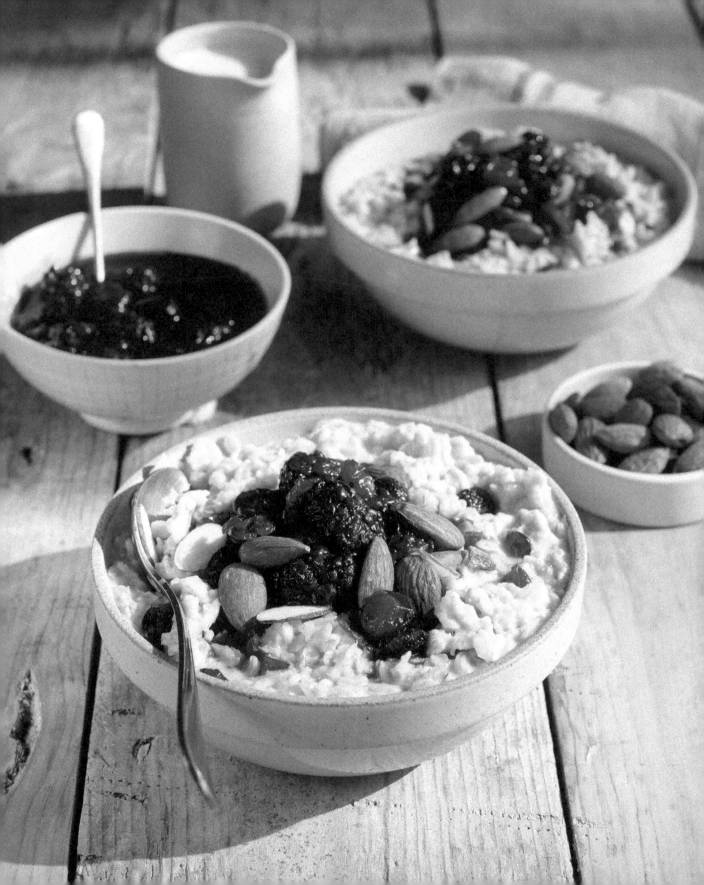

chapter 2
Breakfast

Steel-Cut Oatmeal with Cranberries and Almonds . . . 22

Ginger-Oatmeal Muffins . . . 23

Apple-Cinnamon French Toast Cups . . . 24

Congee with Eggs and Spinach . . . 25

Hard-Cooked Eggs Two Ways . . . 26

Eggs "en Cocotte" . . . 29

Spanish Tortilla . . . 31

Chorizo and Green Chile Breakfast Casserole . . . 32

Tomato, Mozzarella, and Basil Quiche . . . 34

Savory Ham and Cheese Egg Cups . . . 35

*Steel-Cut Oatmeal with Cranberries
and Almonds, page 22*

Steel-Cut Oatmeal with Cranberries and Almonds

Nutty, creamy steel-cut oats get an extra kick from tangy cranberries and toasted nuts in this easy recipe. If you're rushed in the morning, make this the night before and refrigerate it, then reheat and top with the nuts for a warm, filling breakfast.

SERVES 2

PREP & FINISHING:
5 MINUTES

SAUTÉ:
4 MINUTES

PRESSURE COOK:
10 MINUTES HIGH

RELEASE:
NATURAL
10 MINUTES,
THEN QUICK

TOTAL TIME:
40 MINUTES

Per Serving
Calories: 218; Fat: 14 g;
Carbohydrates: 17 g;
Fiber: 3 g; Protein: 6 g;
Sodium: 144 mg

1 tablespoon unsalted butter
½ cup steel-cut oats
Pinch kosher salt
2 teaspoons sugar
1 cup water
½ cup whole milk
¼ teaspoon vanilla extract
¼ cup dried cranberries
¼ cup toasted chopped or whole almonds

1. Select Sauté and adjust to Medium heat. Add the butter to the inner pot. When the butter has melted and stopped foaming, add the oats and stir to coat with the butter. Continue cooking for 2 to 3 minutes, or until the oats have a nutty aroma.

2. Add the salt, sugar, water, milk, vanilla, and cranberries. Stir to combine.

3. Lock the lid into place. Select Pressure Cook or Manual, and adjust the pressure to High and the time to 10 minutes. After cooking, let the pressure release naturally for 10 minutes, then quick release any remaining pressure.

4. Unlock the lid. Spoon the oatmeal into two bowls and top with the almonds. Adjust to your taste, adding extra milk or sugar if you like.

Double It: Oatmeal is a great recipe for doubling, since the leftovers keep well for a couple of days in the refrigerator. Double all the ingredients and increase the salt to ¼ teaspoon. Cook time remains the same.

Make It Dairy-Free: Use a neutral vegetable oil or coconut oil to toast the oats, and replace the whole milk with a plant-based milk or more water.

Ginger-Oatmeal Muffins

Dense and moist, these ginger-laced muffins make a hearty start to the morning. They're portable as well, so you can take an extra one for a midafternoon snack. Not a fan of ginger? Leave it out and just double the amount of cinnamon. If you're a raisin lover, feel free to add them.

1 large egg

¼ cup plain Greek yogurt

¼ cup brown sugar

3 tablespoons unsalted butter, melted

½ teaspoon vanilla extract

⅓ cup quick oats

½ cup all-purpose flour

½ teaspoon baking powder

¼ teaspoon baking soda

½ teaspoon ground ginger

½ teaspoon cinnamon

Pinch kosher salt

2 tablespoons finely chopped crystalized ginger

Nonstick cooking spray

MAKES 4 MUFFINS

PREP & FINISHING:
10 MINUTES

PRESSURE COOK:
12 MINUTES HIGH

RELEASE:
NATURAL
10 MINUTES,
THEN QUICK

TOTAL TIME:
45 MINUTES,
PLUS 10 MINUTES
TO COOL

Per Serving (1 muffin)
Calories: 276; Fat: 11 g;
Carbohydrates: 39 g;
Fiber: 1 g; Protein: 6 g;
Sodium: 207 mg

1. In a medium bowl, stir together the egg, yogurt, brown sugar, butter, and vanilla. In a separate medium bowl, whisk together the oats, flour, baking powder, baking soda, ginger, cinnamon, and salt. Add this to the wet ingredients and stir just until combined. Gently stir in the crystalized ginger.

2. With the cooking spray, generously coat the bottom and sides of four ramekins or custard cups. Pour the batter into the prepared cups, filling them no more than three-quarters full. Cover the cups with aluminum foil.

3. Add 1 cup of water to the inner pot. Place a trivet with handles in the pot and then place the cups on top, stacking them if necessary. Lock the lid into place. Select Pressure Cook or Manual, and adjust the pressure to High and the time to 12 minutes. When cooking is complete, let the pressure release naturally for 10 minutes, then quick release any remaining pressure.

4. Unlock the lid and remove the custard cups. Remove the foil and let the muffins cool for 10 minutes, then run a knife around the edges. Invert the cups to release the muffins.

Use It Up: You can use any remaining chopped crystalized ginger in Coconut-Vanilla Rice Pudding (page 147) or add a tablespoon to the batter for the Carrot Cake (page 154).

Apple-Cinnamon French Toast Cups

These tasty little cups deliver the flavor of French toast crossed with an apple fritter, without the mess of frying. And once they go into the Instant Pot®, you can continue with your morning routine until it's time for breakfast.

SERVES 2

PREP & FINISHING:
12 MINUTES

PRESSURE COOK:
8 MINUTES HIGH

RELEASE:
NATURAL
5 MINUTES,
THEN QUICK

TOTAL TIME:
35 MINUTES

Per Serving
Calories: 217; Fat: 11 g;
Carbohydrates: 23 g;
Fiber: 2 g; Protein: 7 g;
Sodium: 267 mg

Nonstick cooking spray
1 large egg
½ cup whole milk
2 tablespoons heavy (whipping) cream
¼ teaspoon vanilla extract
2 teaspoons brown sugar
¼ teaspoon ground cinnamon
Pinch kosher salt
2 cups bread cubes, cut into ¾-inch pieces (4 to 5 slices)
½ small apple, cored, peeled, and grated

1. With the cooking spray, coat the bottoms and sides of two small ramekins or custard cups.

2. In a medium bowl, whisk the egg thoroughly. Add the milk, cream, vanilla, brown sugar, cinnamon, and salt, and whisk to combine. Add the bread cubes and gently stir to coat with the egg mixture. Let sit for 2 to 3 minutes to let the bread absorb some of the custard. Add the apple and gently stir again. Spoon the bread mixture evenly into the cups. Cover the cups with aluminum foil.

3. Add 1 cup of water to the inner pot. Place a trivet in the pot and then place the ramekins on top. Lock the lid into place. Select Steam and adjust the pressure to High and the time to 8 minutes. After cooking, let the pressure release naturally for 5 minutes, then quick release any remaining pressure.

4. Unlock the lid. Use tongs to remove the ramekins and let cool for several minutes before serving.

Double It: This is an easy recipe to double, though you may need to stack the ramekins, or cook in two batches. If you use two larger ramekins, increase the cook time by 3 or 4 minutes.

Use It Up: The extra half an apple can be used to make Small-Batch Applesauce (page 166).

Congee with Eggs and Spinach

Congee, or rice porridge, is a common breakfast in much of Asia. It's warm and comforting on a cold morning, and just the thing if you're feeling a bit under the weather. This version is thickened with eggs, but the congee is also tasty without them if you want to make this vegan.

⅔ cup arborio or jasmine rice

2 scallions, sliced, green and white parts separated

2 teaspoons minced fresh ginger

2 garlic cloves, minced (about 2 teaspoons)

⅛ teaspoon red pepper flakes

2 tablespoons soy sauce

1 teaspoon rice vinegar (or any wine vinegar)

4 cups low-sodium vegetable or chicken stock

3 cups baby spinach

2 large eggs, beaten

1. Add the rice into the inner pot. Add the white scallion parts, ginger, garlic, red pepper flakes, soy sauce, vinegar, and stock.

2. Lock the lid into place. Select Pressure Cook or Manual, and adjust the pressure to High and the time to 20 minutes. When cooking is complete, let the pressure release naturally for 10 minutes, then quick release any remaining pressure.

3. Unlock the lid. The rice should be soft and the broth should be thick. Add the spinach and scallion greens, and stir until the greens are wilted. Drizzle in the beaten eggs. Stir after adding the eggs if you want threads of cooked egg throughout the broth; whisk constantly while adding the eggs if you want the eggs to thicken and bind with the broth.

Double It: If you have a 6-quart Instant Pot®, you can easily double the recipe (leftovers are great warmed up). The cook time remains the same.

Make It Gluten-Free: Use a gluten-free tamari instead of regular soy sauce.

Use It Up: Use leftover spinach in Minestrone (page 74) or the Artichoke and Spinach Risotto (page 82).

SERVES 2

PREP & FINISHING:
10 MINUTES

PRESSURE COOK:
20 MINUTES HIGH

RELEASE:
NATURAL
10 MINUTES,
THEN QUICK

TOTAL TIME:
50 MINUTES

Per Serving
Calories: 349; Fat: 7 g;
Carbohydrates: 57 g;
Fiber: 4 g; Protein: 15 g;
Sodium: 2566 mg

Hard-Cooked Eggs Two Ways

There's a reason why recipes for hard cooking eggs under pressure vary so widely. So many variables can change the cooking time, from the temperature of the eggs or the water to your particular machine to—believe it or not—the height of the trivet you use. This is what works for me, but if you want to make sure the yolks are completely dry and pale yellow, you may wish to add a minute to the steaming time.

SERVES 2

PREP & FINISHING:
10 MINUTES

PRESSURE COOK:
4 MINUTES HIGH

RELEASE:
QUICK

TOTAL TIME:
25 MINUTES

Per Serving
(avocado toast)
Calories: 358; Fat: 24 g;
Carbohydrates: 20 g;
Fiber: 8 g; Protein: 18 g;
Sodium: 461 mg

Per Serving
(creamy peppered eggs)
Calories: 271; Fat: 24 g;
Carbohydrates: 1 g;
Fiber: 0 g; Protein: 13 g;
Sodium: 217 mg

For the hard-cooked eggs

4 large eggs, at refrigerator
temperature

For egg and avocado toast

1 ripe Hass avocado

1 teaspoon freshly squeezed
lemon juice

½ teaspoon kosher salt

¼ teaspoon smoked paprika

2 large toast slices

For creamy peppered eggs

1 tablespoon heavy
(whipping) cream

2 tablespoons unsalted butter,
at room temperature

½ teaspoon kosher salt

½ teaspoon coarsely ground
black pepper

To hard cook the eggs

1. Fill a medium bowl about halfway with cold water. Add several handfuls of ice cubes. Set aside.

2. Add 1 cup of water to the pot and place the trivet or a steamer basket in the pot. Place the eggs on the trivet. Lock the lid in place. Select Steam and adjust the pressure to High and the time to 4 minutes. After cooking, quick release the pressure. Unlock the lid and use tongs to remove the eggs to the ice bath.

To make egg and avocado toast

1. Let the eggs chill for 5 to 6 minutes.

2. While the eggs cook and cool, cut the avocado in half and remove the pit. Scoop the flesh from the avocado halves into a medium bowl and add the lemon juice, salt, and paprika.

3. When the eggs are cool, peel them and cut them into quarters. Use a large fork or potato masher to break up the eggs and avocados into a coarse mixture. Adjust the seasoning and spread onto the toast slices.

To make creamy peppered eggs

1. Dip the eggs into the ice bath for 30 to 40 seconds, or until just cool enough to handle.

2. Pour the cream into a small bowl and add the butter, salt, and pepper.

3. Peel the eggs and coarsely dice them. Add the eggs to the cream and butter, and stir to melt the butter and coat the eggs. Serve with toast, if you like.

Mini Modification: You may find the eggs slightly overcooked in the Mini, since it takes longer to come to pressure. Start with 4 minutes as the recipe indicates; if you see any hint of green or gray around the yolk, decrease the time to 3 minutes the next time you hard cook eggs.

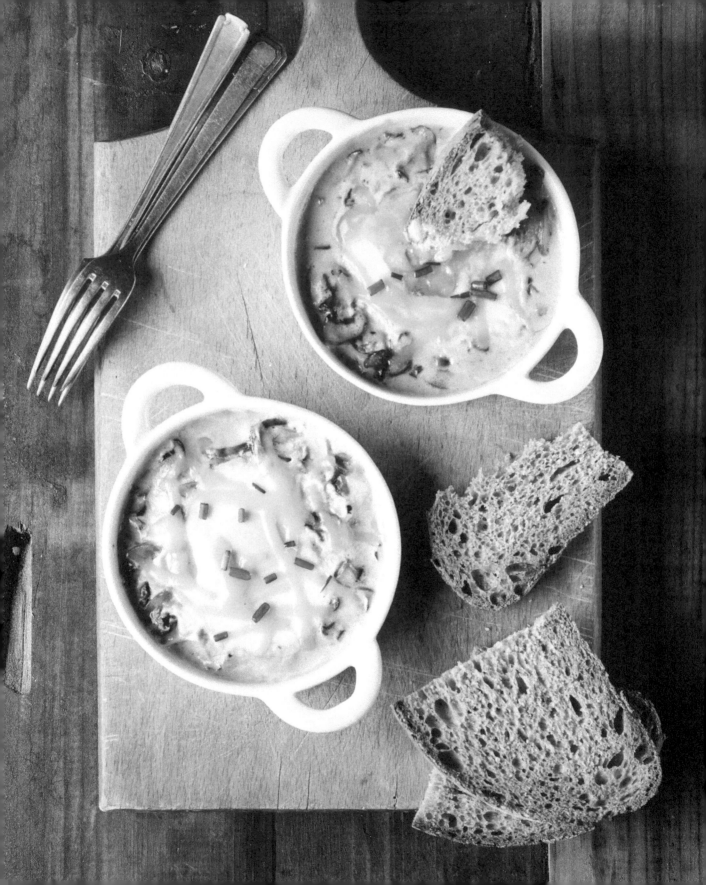

Eggs "en Cocotte"

Eggs en cocotte *is just a fancy term for eggs steamed in cups. They are often flavored with herbs and topped with cheese or cream. This recipe (with a few adaptations) comes from my friend Kerry Beal, who adapted it from* The Art of Living According to Joe Beef: A Cookbook of Sorts.

1 tablespoon unsalted butter

1 teaspoon extra-virgin olive oil

4 white button or cremini mushrooms, halved and sliced

1 tablespoon chopped onion

½ cup vegetable or Mushroom Stock (page 159)

½ cup heavy (whipping) cream

1 tablespoon dry sherry

½ teaspoon kosher salt

Pinch freshly ground black pepper

2 large eggs

2 tablespoons grated sharp Cheddar cheese

1 tablespoon chopped fresh chives (to garnish)

1. Select Sauté and adjust to Medium heat. Add the butter and olive oil to the inner pot and heat until the butter is foaming. Add the mushrooms and cook, stirring occasionally, until they release their liquid, about 5 minutes. Add the onion and cook for about 4 minutes, or until soft.

2. Add the stock, cream, and sherry, and cook until the liquid has reduced by half, about 5 minutes. Stir in the salt and pepper.

3. Divide the mixture between two ramekins. Break an egg into each of the ramekins, and sprinkle each with the Cheddar cheese.

4. Rinse out the inner pot and return it to the base. Add 1 cup of water to the inner pot and place the trivet inside. Place the ramekins, uncovered, on the trivet. ➤

SERVES 2

PREP & FINISHING:
5 MINUTES

SAUTE:
14 MINUTES

PRESSURE COOK:
2 MINUTES HIGH

RELEASE:
QUICK

TOTAL TIME:
30 MINUTES

Per Serving
Calories: 393; Fat: 38 g;
Carbohydrates: 5 g;
Fiber: 0 g; Protein: 10 g;
Sodium: 348 mg

5. Lock the lid into place. Select Pressure Cook or Manual, and adjust the pressure to High and the time to 2 minutes (for runny yolks). After cooking, quick release the pressure.

6. Let the egg cups cool for a minute, and serve garnished with the chives.

Time Saver: You can buy sliced fresh mushrooms at most markets; just remember that they won't last as long as whole mushrooms, so you'll need to use them within a couple of days.

Use It Up: Use leftover mushrooms in Creamy Mushroom-Barley Soup (page 70), Polenta with Mushroom Sauce (page 78), or Shrimp and Grits (page 98). Keep the extra chives to garnish the Curried Cauliflower Soup (page 76).

Spanish Tortilla

In Spain, a tortilla is a flat omelet filled with potatoes, usually cut into wedges and served at room temperature as part of a tapas (small plates) assortment. But it's great for a weekend brunch, served warm with a tangy salad. This version gives you a head start by using frozen hash browns, so they don't have to be cooked for long before you assemble the tortilla.

Nonstick cooking spray

2 tablespoons extra-virgin olive oil

¼ cup chopped onion

1 cup frozen hash browns, thawed

1 teaspoon kosher salt, divided

4 large eggs

1 tablespoon whole milk

1 teaspoon smoked or regular paprika

SERVES 2

PREP & FINISHING:
10 MINUTES

SAUTÉ:
5 MINUTES

PRESSURE COOK:
7 MINUTES HIGH

RELEASE:
NATURAL
8 MINUTES,
THEN QUICK

TOTAL TIME:
40 MINUTES

Per Serving
Calories: 485; Fat: 34 g;
Carbohydrates: 30 g;
Fiber: 3 g; Protein: 16 g;
Sodium: 773 mg

1. With the cooking spray, generously coat the bottom and sides of a 6-inch baking pan or pie pan.

2. Select Sauté and adjust to Medium heat. Add the olive oil and heat until it shimmers. Add the chopped onions. Cook, stirring, for 3 to 4 minutes, or until softened. Stir in the hash browns and ½ teaspoon of salt. Cook for 1 minute, or until heated through. Spoon the potato mixture into the prepared baking pan. Rinse out the inner pot, scraping off any browned bits.

3. In a medium bowl, whisk the eggs until the yolks and whites are completely mixed. Whisk in the milk, paprika, and remaining ½ teaspoon of salt. Pour the egg mixture over the potato mixture.

4. Add 1 cup of water to the inner pot. Place a trivet with handles in the pot and then place the pan on top. Place a piece of aluminum foil over the pan but don't crimp it down. Lock the lid into place. Select Steam and adjust the pressure to High and the time to 7 minutes. After cooking, let the pressure release naturally for 8 minutes, then quick release any remaining pressure.

5. Unlock the lid. Remove the pan and foil. Let cool for 2 to 3 minutes before serving.

Make It Dairy-Free: Replace the milk with water.

Time Saver: Mix the custard while the onions cook and potatoes heat.

Chorizo and Green Chile Breakfast Casserole

Spicy Mexican sausage, cheese, and green chiles enliven this breakfast casserole. The recipe calls for stale bread, which makes it a great way to use up those few slices past their prime. If you're starting with fresh bread, just lay the slices out on a rack for 20 minutes or so (you can do that while you're prepping the remaining ingredients).

SERVES 2

PREP & FINISHING:
10 MINUTES

SAUTÉ:
4 MINUTES

PRESSURE COOK:
12 MINUTES HIGH

RELEASE:
NATURAL
10 MINUTES,
THEN QUICK

TOTAL TIME:
45 MINUTES

Per Serving
Calories: 905; Fat: 62 g;
Carbohydrates: 32 g;
Fiber: 5 g; Protein: 52 g;
Sodium: 1934 mg

½ pound Mexican chorizo, removed from casings if necessary

3 large eggs

¾ cup whole milk

½ teaspoon kosher salt

2 cups stale bread cubes, cut into 1-inch pieces (3 to 4 slices)

1 small (4-ounce) can chopped green chiles, drained and rinsed

½ cup grated Monterey Jack cheese or shredded Mexican blend

Nonstick cooking spray

1. Select Sauté and adjust to Medium heat. Add the chorizo, breaking it up with a spatula into small bite-size pieces. Cook, stirring, until browned. Remove the chorizo and set aside. Rinse out the inner pot, scraping off any browned bits.

2. In a medium bowl, whisk the eggs until the yolks and whites are completely mixed. Whisk in the milk and salt. Add the bread cubes and gently stir to coat with the egg mixture. Let sit for 2 to 3 minutes to let the bread absorb some of the custard, then gently stir again. Add the chorizo, green chiles, and cheese, and gently stir to combine with the bread.

3. With the cooking spray, coat the bottom and sides of a 1-quart baking dish. Add the bread mixture to the baking dish and place a square of aluminum foil over the top. Do not crimp it down as the casserole will expand as it cooks; you just want to keep moisture off the top.

4. Add 1 cup of water to the inner pot. Place a trivet with handles in the pot and then place the baking dish on top. Lock the lid into place. Select Steam and adjust the pressure to High and the time to 12 minutes. After cooking, let the pressure release naturally for 10 minutes, then quick release any remaining pressure.

5. Unlock the lid and carefully remove the casserole from the pot. It should be moist, but a knife inserted in the center should come out with no liquid egg. If it's not done, return it to the pot and put the lid on, but don't turn it on. The residual heat should finish the cooking in 2 to 3 minutes. Let cool for a few minutes, then serve.

6. If you like, you can sprinkle more cheese over the top and run the casserole under the broiler to crisp the top.

Make Ahead: You can prepare the casserole through step 3 the night before and refrigerate it. It will be a bit more custard-like but still delicious. Increase the cook time by 2 minutes when it's straight out of the refrigerator.

Use It Up: Reserve the extra chorizo for the Pinto Beans with Chorizo (page 58). Use the extra cheese in the Creamy Salsa Verde Chicken (page 105).

Tomato, Mozzarella, and Basil Quiche

While you don't get a crisp crust on a pressure-cooked quiche; the trade-off is an exceptionally creamy texture and a much quicker cooking time. With its layered tomatoes, cheese, and herbs, this recipe takes its inspiration from the Italian caprese salad.

SERVES 2

PREP & FINISHING:
10 MINUTES

PRESSURE COOK:
10 MINUTES HIGH

RELEASE:
NATURAL
10 MINUTES,
THEN QUICK

TOTAL TIME:
40 MINUTES

Per Serving
Calories: 457; Fat: 37 g;
Carbohydrates: 7 g;
Fiber: 1 g; Protein: 25 g;
Sodium: 332 mg

1 medium tomato, seeded and diced
¾ teaspoon kosher salt, divided
2 large eggs
⅓ cup whole milk
⅓ cup heavy (whipping) cream
⅛ teaspoon freshly ground black pepper
Nonstick cooking spray
3 ounces grated mozzarella cheese (about 1¼ cups)
2 tablespoons chopped fresh basil

1. In a small strainer placed over a bowl, toss the diced tomato with ¼ teaspoon of salt. Set aside to drain.

2. In a medium bowl, whisk the eggs until the yolks and whites are completely mixed. Add the milk, cream, pepper, and remaining ½ teaspoon of salt and whisk to combine.

3. Coat the bottom and sides of a 1-quart baking dish with the cooking spray. Sprinkle half the cheese over the bottom of the dish. Top with the tomatoes and basil, then add the remaining cheese. Carefully pour the custard over the cheese. Cover the dish with a square of aluminum foil. Do not crimp it down as the quiche will expand as it cooks; you just want to keep moisture off the top.

4. Add 1 cup of water to the inner pot. Place a trivet in the pot and then place the baking dish on top. Lock the lid into place. Select Steam and adjust the pressure to High and the time to 10 minutes. After cooking, let the pressure release naturally for 10 minutes, then quick release any remaining pressure.

5. Unlock the lid. Remove the quiche and let it cool and set for about 10 minutes before slicing and serving.

Use It Up: Use the extra basil in the Warm Thai-Style Green Bean and Tomato Salad (page 50), Rotini with Creamy Basil and Sun-Dried Tomato Sauce (page 81), Italian Tuna and Bean Salad (page 102), or Thai Red Curry Beef (page 129).

Savory Ham and Cheese Egg Cups

A little eggier than quiche, these egg cups are loosely based on the sous vide egg bites popular at Starbucks. My version makes bites a little larger than the Starbucks version, so that each one makes a quick, light breakfast. You can add bacon or cooked vegetables instead of ham, and any cheese you like instead of the Gruyère.

2 large eggs

¼ cup ricotta cheese

2 tablespoons sour cream

¼ teaspoon Dijon-style mustard

¼ teaspoon kosher salt

Pinch freshly ground black or white pepper

Nonstick cooking spray

¼ cup grated Gruyère or other Swiss-style cheese

1 ounce ham, chopped (about 2 tablespoons)

SERVES 2

PREP & FINISHING:
10 MINUTES

PRESSURE COOK:
7 MINUTES HIGH

RELEASE:
NATURAL
5 MINUTES,
THEN QUICK

TOTAL TIME:
35 MINUTES

Per Serving
Calories: 217; Fat: 15 g;
Carbohydrates: 4 g;
Fiber: 0 g; Protein: 16 g;
Sodium: 417 mg

1. In a small bowl, crack the eggs. Add the ricotta, sour cream, mustard, salt, and pepper, and beat with a hand mixer until the mixture is well mixed—no clumps of ricotta or streaks of egg should remain.

2. With the cooking spray, generously spray two ramekins. Place about 1 tablespoon of Gruyère cheese in the bottom of each ramekin and top each with the ham. Pour the egg mixture into the ramekins, dividing it as evenly as possible. Sprinkle each with the remaining cheese. Cover each of the cups with a square of aluminum foil, but do not crimp it around the sides.

3. Add 1 cup of water to the inner pot. Place the trivet inside and then place the ramekins on top. Lock the lid into place. Select Pressure Cook or Manual, and adjust the pressure to High and the time to 7 minutes. After cooking, let the pressure release naturally for 5 minutes, then quick release any remaining pressure.

4. Unlock the lid. Use tongs to remove the ramekins. Let cool for several minutes to let them set completely, then serve.

Use It Up: Use the rest of the ricotta cheese in the Mixed-Up Lasagna (page 133) or the Ricotta Cheesecakes with Balsamic Strawberries (page 152). Extra ham can go in the Ham and Potato Soup (page 140).

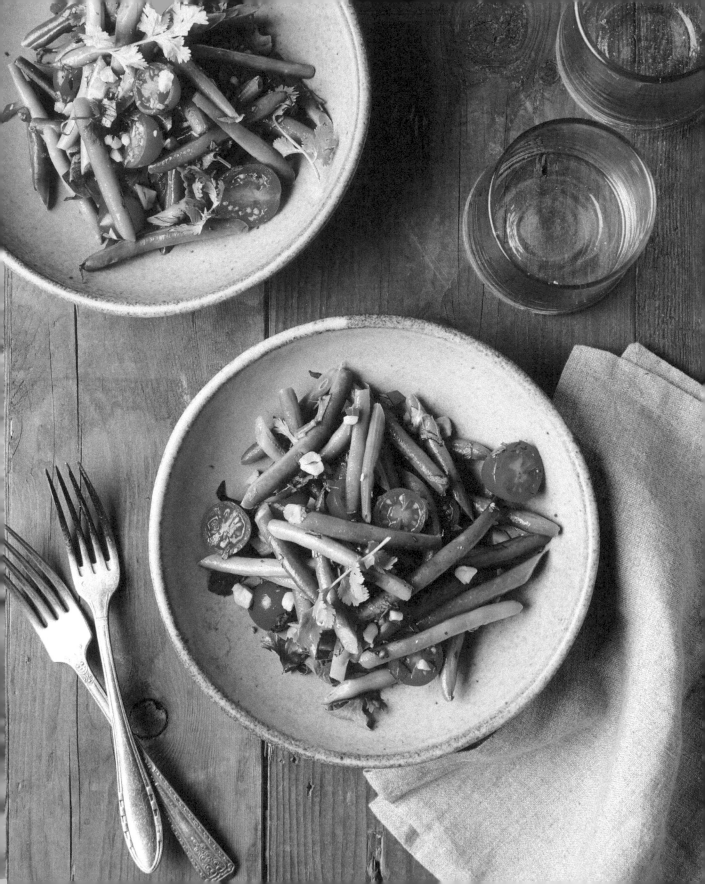

chapter 3
Vegetables and Sides

Crispy Salt and Vinegar Potatoes . . . 38

German Potato Salad . . . 40

Browned Butter Risotto . . . 42

Pimiento Cheese Corn Pudding . . . 43

Beet Salad with Creamy Dill Dressing . . . 44

Tangy Carrot and Celery Salad . . . 45

Roasted Sweet Potatoes and Beets with Rosemary . . . 46

Smashed Red Potatoes with Bacon . . . 48

Asparagus with Balsamic and Pine Nuts . . . 49

Warm Thai-Style Green Bean and Tomato Salad . . . 50

Broccoli Rabe with Lemon-Anchovy Vinaigrette . . . 52

Butter-Braised Cabbage and Carrots . . . 53

*Warm Thai-Style Green Bean
and Tomato Salad, page 50*

Crispy Salt and Vinegar Potatoes

These crisp potato gems are based on a recipe from America's Test Kitchen. The amount of salt might seem alarming, but it seasons the potatoes perfectly throughout. Using the Instant Pot® for the initial cooking saves time and allows you to prep all the other ingredients without having to monitor the potatoes.

SERVES 2

PREP & FINISHING:
35 MINUTES

PRESSURE COOK:
5 MINUTES HIGH

RELEASE:
QUICK

TOTAL TIME:
50 MINUTES

Per Serving
Calories: 317; Fat: 25 g;
Carbohydrates: 22 g;
Fiber: 3 g; Protein: 2 g;
Sodium: 2235 mg

1 quart hot tap water
5 ounces salt (about ½ cup fine salt or 1 cup kosher salt)
10 ounces small (about 1½ inches in diameter) red or gold potatoes

¼ cup extra-virgin olive oil
2 tablespoons malt or other vinegar, divided

1. Preheat the oven to 400°F.

2. Add the hot water to the inner pot and add the salt, stirring to dissolve. Add the potatoes.

3. Lock the lid into place. Select Pressure Cook or Manual, and adjust the pressure to High and the time to 5 minutes. After cooking, quick release the pressure.

4. Unlock the lid. Pour the potatoes into a colander to drain. Let them cool for 10 minutes.

5. While the potatoes cool, generously coat a small baking sheet or sheet pan with about half of the olive oil, reserving the rest for steps 6 and 7. Place the cooled potatoes, spaced evenly, on the sheet. Use a paring knife, cut a shallow X across the top of each potato (about ¼ inch deep).

6. Coat the bottom of a heavy glass or a heavy spatula with some of the remaining oil. Use the glass or spatula to gently smash the potatoes to about ½-inch thickness. Work carefully so the potatoes don't break into pieces.

7. Brush the tops of the potatoes lightly with oil, then brush with about 1 tablespoon of vinegar. You may not need all the oil, depending on how many potatoes you have.

8. Roast the potatoes for 15 to 20 minutes or until crisp and golden brown. Remove the pan from the oven and brush the potatoes with the remaining 1 tablespoon of vinegar. Serve immediately.

Double It: You can double the amount of potatoes. Keep the water and salt amounts the same, but increase the olive oil and vinegar as needed. Do not crowd the potatoes on the sheet pan; use two if necessary, and rotate them halfway through roasting.

German Potato Salad

Unlike its American counterpart, German Potato salad is served warm, with bacon and a slightly sweet vinaigrette instead of a creamy dressing. For a tangier salad, you can replace the mustard seeds with a couple teaspoons of whole-grain mustard.

9 ounces small (2-inch) red potatoes

3 tablespoons cider vinegar, divided

¼ teaspoon kosher salt, plus more as needed

1 tablespoon vegetable oil

1 or 2 bacon slices, chopped (about ⅓ cup)

⅓ cup chopped onion

¼ cup chopped celery

1½ teaspoons sugar

¼ teaspoon mustard seeds or mustard powder

¼ teaspoon celery seeds

1 tablespoon chopped parsley

SERVES 2

PREP & FINISHING:
8 MINUTES

PRESSURE COOK:
3 MINUTES HIGH

RELEASE:
QUICK

SAUTÉ:
7 MINUTES

TOTAL TIME:
30 MINUTES

Per Serving
Calories: 283; Fat: 15 g;
Carbohydrates: 26 g;
Fiber: 4 g; Protein: 10 g;
Sodium: 407 mg

1. Trim and slice the potatoes about ¼ inch thick. Cut the slices in half. Arrange the potatoes in a steamer basket as evenly as possible.

2. Add 1 cup of water to the inner pot and place the steamer basket inside. Lock the lid into place. Select Steam and adjust the pressure to High and the time to 3 minutes. After cooking, quick release the pressure.

3. Unlock the lid. Remove the steamer basket from the pot. Transfer the potatoes to a bowl and sprinkle with 1 tablespoon of vinegar and the salt. Toss gently and set aside.

4. Empty the pot, dry it, and return it to the base.

5. Select Sauté and adjust to High heat. Add the vegetable oil. Add the bacon and cook, stirring often, for about 4 minutes, or until it's mostly crisp and the fat has rendered. Remove the bacon to a paper towel–lined plate.

6. Add the onion and celery, and stir to coat with the fat. Cook for 1 minute, then press Cancel to turn off the heat. Add the remaining 2 tablespoons of vinegar, sugar, mustard seeds, and celery seeds. Stir to dissolve the sugar.

7. Pour the dressing over the potatoes and add the reserved bacon and parsley. Toss gently and taste, adding salt as necessary.

Double It: Double all the ingredients (except the water for steaming). The larger amount of bacon will take longer to cook, but the time under pressure remains the same.

Easier Together: One of you can prep and cook the potatoes while the other dices the bacon and vegetables.

Browned Butter Risotto

Most people think of risotto as a main dish, but it also makes a wonderful accompaniment to simple roasted or grilled steak, chicken, or pork chops. Let the risotto cook while you get the rest of dinner together, and you'll have the most elegant of meals in no time—even on a weeknight!

SERVES 2

PREP & FINISHING:
10 MINUTES

SAUTÉ:
6 MINUTES

PRESSURE COOK:
8 MINUTES HIGH

RELEASE:
QUICK

TOTAL TIME:
35 MINUTES

Per Serving
Calories: 313; Fat: 19 g;
Carbohydrates: 27 g;
Fiber: 1 g; Protein: 5 g;
Sodium: 386 mg

3 tablespoons unsalted butter

1 tablespoon chopped shallot or onion

⅓ cup arborio rice

3 tablespoons dry white wine, such as Sauvignon Blanc

1¼ cups low-sodium chicken stock

¼ teaspoon kosher salt

½ ounce (about ¼ cup) finely shredded Parmesan cheese

1. Select Sauté and adjust to Medium heat. Add the butter. Once melted, continue to cook until the milk solids begin to brown, 3 to 5 minutes. Pour the butter out of the pot into a small dish or bowl. Return 1 tablespoon to the pot, setting aside the remaining 2 tablespoons.

2. Add the shallot and cook, stirring often, for 1 to 2 minutes, or until it begins to soften. Add the rice and stir to coat the grains with the butter.

3. Add the wine and bring it to a simmer. Let the wine mostly evaporate, then add the stock and salt. Stir to combine.

4. Lock the lid into place. Select Pressure Cook or Manual, and adjust the pressure to High and the time to 8 minutes. After cooking, quick release the pressure.

5. Unlock the lid. Test the risotto; the rice should be soft with a slightly firm center and the sauce should be creamy. If it's not quite done or it's too soupy, select Sauté and simmer for 1 to 2 minutes. Stir in the cheese and serve.

Use It Up: Extra arborio rice can be used in the Congee with Eggs and Spinach (page 25) or the main dish Artichoke and Spinach Risotto (page 82).

Pimiento Cheese Corn Pudding

Many years ago, a friend of mine made a delicious, creamy corn pudding as a side for dinner. I didn't think to ask for the recipe, but a few months ago, I wanted to create something similar. It turns out that most of what's called "corn pudding" is really just moist cornbread. So I developed this recipe, which adds the flavors of pimiento cheese to the creamy corn. If you can find roasted piquillo peppers in a jar, they're perfect for this recipe, but regular jarred roasted red peppers work well, too.

2 teaspoons all-purpose flour
½ teaspoon sugar
½ teaspoon baking powder
¼ teaspoon kosher salt
1 large egg
⅓ cup heavy (whipping) cream
1 tablespoon unsalted butter, melted and cooled
3 ounces sharp Cheddar cheese, grated (about 1 cup)

1 cup frozen corn kernels, thawed
¼ cup chopped roasted red pepper
1 tablespoon finely chopped onion
½ teaspoon hot pepper sauce, such as Tabasco
Nonstick cooking spray

PSERVES 2

PREP & FINISHING:
10 MINUTES

PRESSURE COOK:
15 MINUTES HIGH

RELEASE:
10 MINUTES
NATURAL,
THEN QUICK

TOTAL TIME:
45 MINUTES

Per Serving
Calories: 486; Fat: 38 g;
Carbohydrates: 22 g;
Fiber: 3 g; Protein: 18 g;
Sodium: 533 mg

1. In a small bowl, stir together the flour, sugar, baking powder, and salt until blended. In a medium bowl, whisk together the egg, cream, and melted butter until blended. Stir the flour mixture into the egg mixture. Stir in the cheese, corn, red pepper, onion, and hot sauce.

2. Generously grease the bottom and sides of a 1-quart-round baking dish. Spoon the mixture into the baking dish and cover with aluminum foil.

3. Add 1 cup of water to the inner pot. Place the trivet inside and then place the baking dish on the trivet. Lock the lid into place. Select Pressure Cook or Manual, and adjust the pressure to High and the time to 15 minutes. After cooking, let the pressure release naturally for 10 minutes, then quick release any remaining pressure.

4. Unlock the lid. Remove the dish from the pot and let sit 2 or 3 minutes before serving.

Beet Salad with Creamy Dill Dressing

I hated beets when I was a kid, which is a shame since my father grew them every year in his garden. I could kick myself now when I think of all the fresh beets I missed back then. I first grew to like them in salads like this one, which I think Dad would have liked.

2 medium (2- to 3-inch) beets, stemmed and roots trimmed

2 teaspoons mayonnaise

1 tablespoon Greek yogurt

¼ teaspoon kosher salt

1 teaspoon freshly squeezed lemon juice

½ teaspoon grated lemon zest

1 tablespoon minced fresh dill

SERVES 2

PREP & FINISHING:
10 MINUTES

PRESSURE COOK:
8 MINUTES HIGH

RELEASE:
NATURAL
6 MINUTES,
THEN QUICK

TOTAL TIME:
35 MINUTES

Per Serving
Calories: 73; Fat: 2 g;
Carbohydrates: 12 g;
Fiber: 2 g; Protein: 3 g;
Sodium: 166 mg

1. Place the beets in the steamer basket. Add 1 cup of water to the inner pot and place the steamer basket inside. Lock the lid into place. Select Pressure Cook or Manual, and adjust pressure to High and the time to 8 minutes. After cooking, let the pressure release naturally for 6 minutes, then quick release any remaining pressure.

2. Unlock the lid. Remove the beets and set aside to cool.

3. While the beets cool, make the dressing. In a medium bowl, whisk together the mayonnaise, yogurt, salt, lemon juice, and lemon zest.

4. When the beets are cool enough to handle, peel them with a paring knife (the skin should just slip off). Cut in half, then slice into large bite-size pieces. Add to the dressing and toss to coat. Just before serving, add the dill and toss again.

Double It: You can easily cook extra beets for more salad or other uses. Use just 1 cup of water for steaming, and peel the beets just when they cool—it's easier that way.

Tangy Carrot and Celery Salad

This recipe falls somewhere between quick pickles and the South American escabeche. It's great with rich dishes like the Ham and Potato Soup (page 140) or served alongside most sandwiches. If you prefer, you can use all carrots or all celery, but I like the combination of the two vegetables best.

2 large carrots, peeled and
   cut into ½-inch rounds
   (about 1 cup)
2 celery ribs, sliced ½ inch thick
   (about 1 cup)
1 tablespoon extra-virgin olive oil

2 tablespoons red wine vinegar
1½ teaspoons sugar
1 teaspoon kosher salt
⅛ teaspoon mustard seeds
⅛ teaspoon celery seeds

1. Place the carrots and celery in a steamer basket. Add 1 cup of water to the inner pot and place the steamer basket inside. Lock the lid into place. Select Steam and adjust pressure to High and the time to 2 minutes. After cooking, quick release the pressure.

2. While the vegetables cook, make the dressing. In a medium bowl, whisk together the olive oil, vinegar, sugar, salt, mustard seeds, and celery seeds.

3. Unlock the lid. Transfer the cooked carrots and celery to the bowl. Let them cool in the dressing, tossing occasionally, for 10 to 15 minutes.

Double It: The salad keeps in the refrigerator for several days, so it's perfect for doubling. Double all the ingredients except the water for steaming. You may not need quite all the dressing.

SERVES 2

PREP & FINISHING:
10 MINUTES

PRESSURE COOK:
2 MINUTES HIGH

RELEASE:
QUICK

TOTAL TIME:
25 MINUTES

Per Serving
Calories: 114; Fat: 7 g;
Carbohydrates: 12 g;
Fiber: 3 g; Protein: 1 g;
Sodium: 683 mg

Roasted Sweet Potatoes and Beets with Rosemary

Beets and sweet potatoes are a great combination, especially roasted. But they're so dense, they take a long time to cook through, and it can be tricky to make sure they don't burn on the outside before the centers are done. Using the Instant Pot® gives you a head start cooking, so the final roasting can be done in a flash.

SERVES 2

PREP & FINISHING:
15 MINUTES

PRESSURE COOK:
6 MINUTES HIGH

RELEASE:
QUICK

TOTAL TIME:
30 MINUTES

Per Serving
Calories: 164; Fat: 7 g;
Carbohydrates: 24 g;
Fiber: 5 g; Protein: 3 g;
Sodium: 204 mg

2 small (2-inch) beets
1 small (about 8 ounces) sweet potato
1 tablespoon extra-virgin olive oil
½ teaspoon kosher salt
2 teaspoons fresh finely chopped rosemary, thyme, or oregano

1. Preheat the oven to 400°F.

2. Cut the beets in half and trim the roots off. Place the beets and sweet potato in a steamer basket or on the trivet. Add 1 cup of water to the inner pot and place the steamer basket inside. Lock the lid into place. Select Pressure Cook or Manual, and adjust pressure to High and the time to 6 minutes. After cooking, quick release the pressure.

3. Unlock the lid. Remove the vegetables and let them cool slightly, then peel and cut into 1-inch chunks. They should be softened, but not completely cooked through. Place them on a baking sheet. Drizzle with the olive oil and sprinkle with the salt. Gently toss to coat.

4. Roast the vegetables for 8 to 10 minutes, or until cooked through and browned in spots on the outside. Remove from the oven and sprinkle with the rosemary. Return to the oven for just a minute to bloom the aroma and flavor of the rosemary, then serve.

Double It: If you want to double the recipe, use the same size vegetables, but twice as many. If you use larger beets and a huge sweet potato, they won't cook evenly in the Instant Pot® and will require more time in the oven.

Use It Up: You can use a couple of rosemary sprigs in the Italian Pork Sandwiches (page 136).

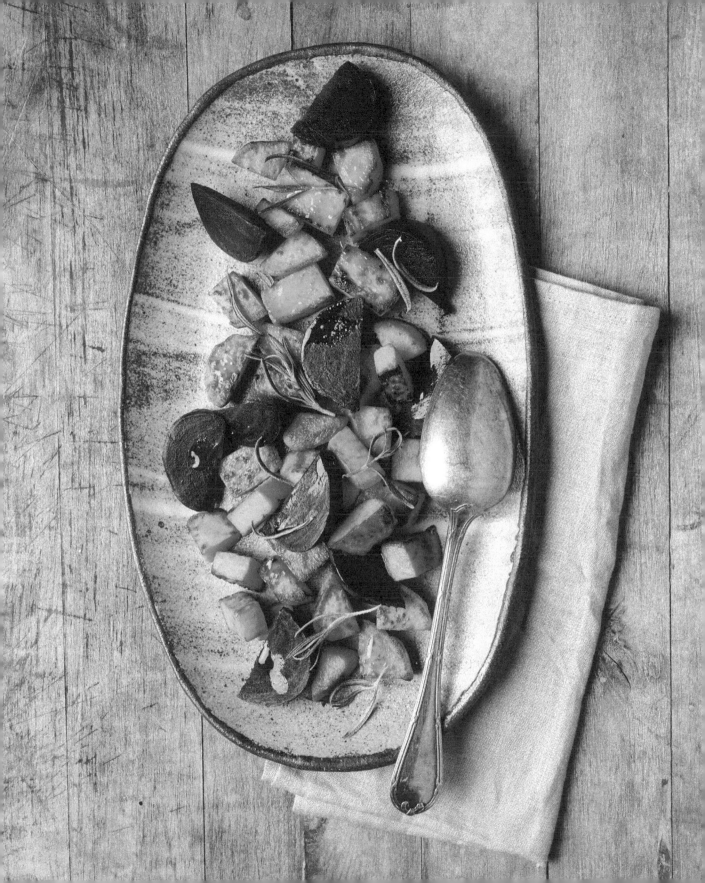

Smashed Red Potatoes with Bacon

One of my favorite ways to prepare red potatoes is to steam them, then smash them lightly with cream and cheese. The only way it gets better is to add bacon. For a fancier version, you can scoop the finished potatoes into a baking dish, top with grated Parmesan cheese, and cook under the broiler until crisp on top.

SERVES 2

PREP & FINISHING:
10 MINUTES

SAUTÉ:
5 MINUTES

PRESSURE COOK:
4 MINUTES HIGH

RELEASE:
QUICK

TOTAL TIME:
30 MINUTES

Per Serving
Calories: 404; Fat: 28 g;
Carbohydrates: 22 g;
Fiber: 3 g; Protein: 17 g;
Sodium: 914 mg

9 ounces red potatoes (1 large or 2 or 3 medium)

¼ teaspoon kosher salt, plus more as needed

3 bacon slices, diced

⅛ teaspoon freshly ground black pepper

¼ cup heavy (whipping) cream, plus more as needed

1 ounce sharp Cheddar cheese, coarsely shredded (about ½ cup)

1 scallion, green part only, chopped

1. Trim and cut the potatoes into 1-inch chunks. Place the potatoes in a steamer basket. Add 1 cup of water to the inner pot and place the steamer basket inside. Lock the lid into place. Select Steam and adjust the pressure to High and the time to 4 minutes. After cooking, quick release the pressure.

2. Unlock the lid. Remove the steamer basket from the pot and sprinkle the potatoes with the salt.

3. Empty the inner pot, dry it, and return it to the base.

4. Select Sauté and adjust to High heat. Add the bacon and cook, stirring, for about 4 minutes, or until it's mostly crisp and the fat has rendered. Transfer the potatoes back to the pot and add the pepper and cream. Use a potato masher to crush the potatoes into the cream, then stir in the cheese. The potatoes should be chunky—too much mashing can make them gluey. Let sit for a few minutes until the cheese is melted, then stir in the scallion.

Double It: This dish is great for company—easy but impressive, especially if you opt for the fancy gratin version with Parmesan cheese and placed under the broiler. Double everything except the water for steaming the potatoes.

Asparagus with Balsamic and Pine Nuts

I tend to like asparagus done simply—roasted, or blanched and tossed in a vinaigrette. This way, flavored with a splash of balsamic vinegar and the crunch of pine nuts, is equally simple. When you buy asparagus, look for thick stalks and fresh looking, firm tips. "Pencil-thin" asparagus comes from the very beginning or end of the growing season and tends to be stringy. This quick and easy recipe cooks the asparagus while the pot comes to pressure.

½ pound asparagus, ends trimmed

1 tablespoon extra-virgin olive oil

¼ teaspoon kosher salt

1 teaspoon balsamic vinegar

1 tablespoon toasted pine nuts

1. Place the asparagus in a steamer basket. Add 1 cup of water to the inner pot and place the steamer basket inside. Lock the lid into place. Select Steam and adjust pressure to High and the time to 0 minutes. After cooking, quick release the pressure.

2. Unlock the lid. Remove the asparagus. Empty the inner pot, dry it, and return it to the base.

3. Select Sauté and adjust to High heat. Add the olive oil and heat until it shimmers. Add the asparagus and salt and cook, stirring often, for 1 to 2 minutes, or until the asparagus is golden brown in spots. Transfer the asparagus to a plate and drizzle with the balsamic vinegar. Top it with the pine nuts.

Make It New: If you buy a whole pound of asparagus, you can steam it all and reserve half. Refrigerate it, and then toss with a vinaigrette for a salad later in the week, or add it to the Italian Tuna and Bean Salad (page 102) or Greek Salad with Bulgur Wheat (page 62).

SERVES 2

PREP & FINISHING:
5 MINUTES

PRESSURE COOK:
0 MINUTES HIGH

RELEASE:
QUICK

SAUTÉ:
2 MINUTES

TOTAL TIME:
15 MINUTES

Per Serving
Calories: 112; Fat: 10 g;
Carbohydrates: 5 g;
Fiber: 3 g; Protein: 3 g;
Sodium: 150 mg

Warm Thai-Style
Green Bean and Tomato Salad

A few years ago, I was searching for a side dish for a Thai-inspired main course, and came across a salad with chopped tomatoes and green beans, garnished with lots of herbs and peanuts. A Thai acquaintance of mine let me know in no uncertain terms that it was not an authentic Thai recipe, since a Thai recipe would never include raw tomatoes. Oh well. It's still really good.

SERVES 2

PREP & FINISHING:
10 MINUTES

PRESSURE COOK:
0 MINUTES HIGH

RELEASE:
QUICK

TOTAL TIME:
20 MINUTES

Per Serving
Calories: 231; Fat: 9 g;
Carbohydrates: 38 g;
Fiber: 9 g; Protein: 8 g;
Sodium: 214 mg

For the salad

6 ounces green beans, washed, trimmed, and cut into 1-inch pieces

¼ teaspoon kosher salt

¾ cup cherry or grape tomatoes, halved

¼ cup chopped cilantro

2 tablespoons chiffonade-cut fresh basil

2 tablespoons chopped roasted cashews

For the dressing

1 small fresh red chile (Fresno or red jalapeño), seeded and finely chopped

2 teaspoons freshly squeezed lime juice

2 teaspoons sugar

2 teaspoons fish sauce

1 small garlic clove, minced or pressed

1. Place the green beans in a steamer basket. Add 1 cup of water to the inner pot and place the steamer basket inside. Lock the lid into place. Select Steam and adjust the pressure to High and the time to 0 minutes.

2. While the pressure builds to cook the beans, make the dressing. In a medium bowl, whisk together all the ingredients.

3. When the beans are cooked, quick release the pressure. Unlock the lid. Remove the beans; they should be mostly tender but should have a slightly crisp center. Sprinkle them with the salt and let cool for a minute. Add the beans to the dressing and add the tomatoes. Toss well with the dressing and let sit for 2 to 3 minutes, or until barely warm. Add the cilantro, basil, and cashews, and toss gently. Serve immediately.

Double It: Cook double the amount of the green beans and use the extra in the Italian Tuna and Bean Salad (page 102).

Use It Up: Use extra cherry tomatoes in the Farfalle with Salmon, Fennel, and Tomatoes (page 92). The rest of the cilantro can go in the Cilantro-Coconut Shrimp and Broccoli (page 100); use the remaining basil in Rotini with Creamy Basil and Sun-Dried Tomato Sauce (page 81).

Broccoli Rabe with Lemon-Anchovy Vinaigrette

Broccoli rabe (rapini in Italian) is related to broccoli but has fewer and smaller florets, longer stems, and lots of leaves—and it's much more bitter. The first time I had it was in an Italian restaurant. It was served steamed and cooled, with a tart, anchovy-laced dressing and shaved Parmigiano over the top. I fell in love with it. If your market is like mine, you'll have to buy a big bunch, but don't worry—you can steam it all and then use the rest in several other recipes.

SERVES 2

PREP & FINISHING:
10 MINUTES

PRESSURE COOK:
0 MINUTES HIGH

RELEASE:
QUICK

TOTAL TIME:
20 MINUTES

Per Serving
Calories: 200; Fat: 20 g;
Carbohydrates: 7 g;
Fiber: 6 g; Protein: 10 g;
Sodium: 445 mg

1 bunch (12 to 16 ounces) broccoli rabe

¼ teaspoon kosher salt

1 tablespoon freshly squeezed lemon juice

1 teaspoon anchovy paste

2 tablespoons extra-virgin olive oil

½ ounce Parmesan cheese, shaved into thin slices or crumbled

1. Cut off and discard the tough ends of the broccoli rabe stems and any brown, wilted leaves. Cut the broccoli rabe into 1½-inch-long pieces.

2. Place the broccoli rabe in a steamer basket. Add 1 cup of water to the inner pot and place the steamer basket inside. Lock the lid into place. Select Steam and adjust the pressure to High and the time to 0 minutes. After cooking, quick release the pressure.

3. Unlock the lid. Remove the broccoli rabe and rinse it with cold water to stop the cooking. Place about a third of it in a medium bowl and sprinkle with the salt. (Blot the rest dry and wrap it loosely in a paper towel, then put it in a plastic bag in the refrigerator.)

4. To make the dressing, pour the lemon juice into a small jar and add the anchovy paste and olive oil. Screw the lid on the jar and shake until well combined. Pour the dressing over the broccoli rabe and toss gently. Divide it between two plates and top with the Parmesan cheese.

Use It Up: Use the remaining broccoli rabe in the White Bean Stew with Broccoli Rabe (page 56), Penne with Italian Sausage and Broccoli Rabe (page 132), or Italian Pork Sandwiches (page 136). Use the anchovy paste in the French Onion Soup Dip Sandwiches (page 126).

Butter-Braised Cabbage and Carrots

Unlike the more typical braised sweet and sour cabbage, this recipe uses green rather than red cabbage, and keeps the cabbage in wedges so it's easier to brown. The sweetness of the carrots is a nice complement to the hearty cabbage. The dish goes well with pork or corned beef.

3 tablespoons unsalted butter

¼ small green cabbage head, core intact, halved

½ small onion, sliced

2 medium carrots, cut into 1-inch chunks

1 teaspoon kosher salt

¼ teaspoon freshly ground black pepper

⅓ cup chicken or vegetable stock

1 tablespoon chopped parsley, for garnish

SERVES 2

PREP & FINISHING:
5 MINUTES

SAUTÉ:
6 MINUTES

PRESSURE COOK:
4 MINUTES HIGH

RELEASE:
QUICK

TOTAL TIME:
25 MINUTES

Per Serving
Calories: 214; Fat: 18 g;
Carbohydrates: 14 g;
Fiber: 5 g; Protein: 2 g;
Sodium: 492 mg

1. Select Sauté and adjust to Medium heat. Add the butter to the inner pot. After it foams, add the cabbage wedges. Let them cook, undisturbed, for 2 to 3 minutes, or until browned in spots. Turn to the other cut side and continue to cook until that side is browned, too. Add the onion and carrots, and stir to coat them with the butter. Sprinkle with the salt and pepper. Pour in the stock.

2. Lock the lid into place. Select Pressure Cook or Manual, and adjust the pressure to High and the time to 4 minutes. After cooking, quick release the pressure.

3. Unlock the lid. Serve the vegetables with the braising liquid spooned over the top and garnished with the parsley.

Make It Dairy-Free: While the butter gives the dish a fabulous flavor, you can also use olive oil for a dairy-free version.

Use It Up: Use the remaining cabbage in the Kielbasa and Vegetable Stew (page 131) or the Barbecue Chicken Sandwiches with Slaw (page 116).

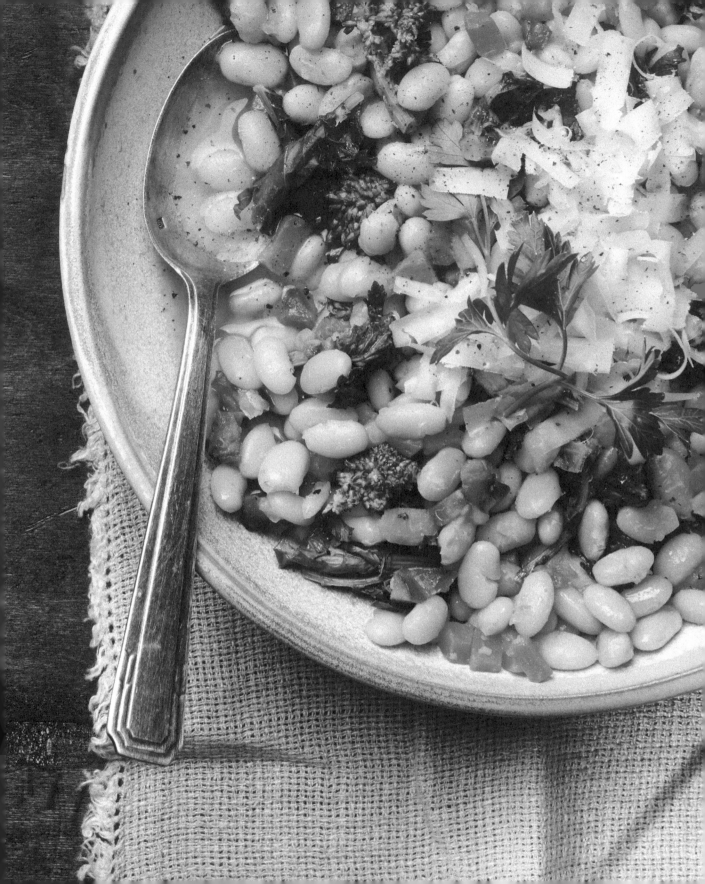

chapter 4
Beans and Grains

White Bean Stew with Broccoli Rabe . . . 56

North African Chickpea Stew . . . 57

Pinto Beans with Chorizo . . . 58

Southwestern Black Bean Salad . . . 60

Brown Rice and Broccoli Cheese Casserole . . . 61

Greek Salad with Bulgur Wheat . . . 62

Rice Pilaf with Bacon and Water Chestnuts . . . 64

Herbed Wild Rice Pilaf with Almonds . . . 66

Lentils with Red Peppers and Feta . . . 67

Jamaican Rice and Peas . . . 68

Creamy Mushroom-Barley Soup . . . 70

Quinoa with Marinated Artichokes and Peppers . . . 71

White Bean Stew with Broccoli Rabe, page 56

White Bean Stew with Broccoli Rabe

Combining beans and greens is a common—and delicious—Italian dinner tradition. In this dish of cannellini beans flavored with ham, broccoli rabe provides color and a hint of bitterness. If you don't have broccoli rabe, you can use chard instead. Sauté it briefly before adding it after the beans pressure cook.

SERVES 2
AS A MAIN DISH

PREP & FINISHING:
10 MINUTES

SAUTÉ:
5 MINUTES

PRESSURE COOK:
12 MINUTES HIGH

RELEASE:
NATURAL
10 MINUTES,
THEN QUICK

TOTAL TIME:
45 MINUTES,
PLUS 8 HOURS
TO SOAK

Per Serving
Calories: 504; Fat: 21 g;
Carbohydrates: 51 g;
Fiber: 23 g; Protein: 33 g;
Sodium: 509 mg

1 quart water
1 tablespoon plus ½ teaspoon
  kosher salt, divided
¼ pound cannellini beans
2 tablespoons extra-virgin olive oil
½ small onion, chopped
1 small carrot, chopped
2 garlic cloves, minced

½ cup diced cooked ham
1 bay leaf
1½ cups low-sodium chicken stock
4 ounces steamed Broccoli Rabe
  (see page 52)
¼ cup grated Parmesan or
  similar cheese
1 tablespoon chopped fresh parsley

1. In a large bowl, dissolve 1 tablespoon of salt in the water. Add the beans and soak at room temperature for 8 to 24 hours. Drain and rinse.

2. Select Sauté and adjust to Medium heat. Add the olive oil to the inner pot and heat until shimmering. Add the onion and carrot and sprinkle with ¼ teaspoon of salt. Cook, stirring often, until the onion pieces separate and soften. Add the garlic and cook for about 1 minute, or until fragrant. Add the drained beans, remaining ¼ teaspoon of salt, ham, bay leaf, and stock.

3. Lock the lid into place. Select Pressure Cook or Manual, and adjust the pressure to High and the time to 12 minutes. After cooking, let the pressure release naturally for 10 minutes, then quick release any remaining pressure.

4. Unlock the lid. Stir in the broccoli rabe and bring to a simmer to heat it through and thicken the sauce slightly. Taste the beans and adjust the seasoning. Ladle into bowls and sprinkle with the cheese and parsley.

Easier Together: If one of you sautés the onion and carrots while the other chops the ham and grates the cheese, you'll save some time.

Use It Up: Extra ham can go in the Ham and Potato Soup (page 140) or the Savory Ham and Cheese Egg Cups (page 35). If you have a whole bunch of broccoli rabe, it's easy to steam it all, then use the remainder in the Penne with Italian Sausage and Broccoli Rabe (page 132) or Italian Pork Sandwiches (page 136).

North African Chickpea Stew

Chickpeas (garbanzo beans) are popular throughout the Middle East and Northern Africa in dishes from hummus to falafel to savory stews like this one. Make it spicy with harissa if you like, or omit it for a milder stew.

1 quart plus 2 cups water, divided

1 tablespoon plus 1 teaspoon kosher salt

½ pound dried chickpeas

3 garlic cloves, minced

1 small onion, chopped

½ (14-ounce) can diced tomatoes

1 teaspoon cumin seeds

1 tablespoon extra-virgin olive oil

Juice of 1 lemon (about 2 tablespoons)

1 tablespoon harissa (optional)

¼ cup Greek yogurt (optional)

SERVES 2

PREP & FINISHING:
10 MINUTES

PRESSURE COOK:
6 MINUTES HIGH

RELEASE:
NATURAL
8 MINUTES,
THEN QUICK

TOTAL TIME:
35 MINUTES,
PLUS 8 HOURS
TO SOAK

Per Serving
Calories: 524; Fat: 14 g;
Carbohydrates: 79 g;
Fiber: 22 g; Protein: 24 g;
Sodium: 324 mg

1. In a large bowl, dissolve 1 tablespoon of salt in 1 quart of water. Add the chickpeas and soak at room temperature for 8 hours to overnight. Drain and rinse the chickpeas.

2. Place the chickpeas in the inner pot. Add the garlic, onion, tomatoes, cumin, olive oil, the remaining 1 teaspoon of salt, and 2 cups of water.

3. Lock the lid into place. Select Pressure Cook or Manual, and adjust the pressure to High and the time to 6 minutes. After cooking, let the pressure release naturally for 8 minutes, then quick release any remaining pressure.

4. Unlock the lid. Taste the soup and adjust the seasoning, if necessary. There should be plenty of broth; if the texture is too thick, add more water. Stir in the lemon juice and harissa (if using). Serve, garnished with the yogurt (if using).

Double It: The stew is wonderful leftover. Use the same amount of water to soak the entire pound of chickpeas. Double all the remaining ingredients and keep the cooking time the same.

Pinto Beans with Chorizo

Mexican chorizo is completely different from the Spanish and Portuguese versions, which are cured. The Mexican style is fresh—sometimes in casings, sometimes in bulk. The flavor is so complex that you hardly need any more seasonings for this easy bean dish. You can top the beans with cheese and salsa and eat the dish like chili, or pile the filling into tortillas for tacos. Either way, it's delicious.

SERVES 2

AS A MAIN DISH

PREP & FINISHING:
5 MINUTES

SAUTÉ:
4 MINUTES

PRESSURE COOK:
12 MINUTES HIGH

RELEASE:
NATURAL
5 MINUTES,
THEN QUICK

TOTAL TIME:
40 MINUTES,
PLUS 8 HOURS
TO SOAK

Per Serving
Calories: 561; Fat: 24 g;
Carbohydrates: 56 g;
Fiber: 13 g; Protein: 32 g;
Sodium: 423 mg

2 cups water

1 tablespoon plus ¼ teaspoon kosher salt, divided

¼ pound pinto beans (about ⅔ cup)

¼ pound Mexican chorizo

1½ cups low-sodium chicken stock

1 small tomato, seeded and diced (or use ¼ cup canned diced tomatoes, drained)

1 tablespoon chopped cilantro

¼ cup grated Monterey jack cheese

2 tablespoons jarred tomatillo salsa (I like Frontera brand)

1. In a large bowl, add the water. Dissolve 1½ teaspoons of salt in the water. Add the beans and soak at room temperature for 8 to 24 hours. Drain and rinse.

2. Select Sauté and adjust to Medium heat. Add the chorizo and cook, stirring often, until it's browned and broken up. Add the drained pinto beans, ¼ teaspoon of salt, and stock.

3. Lock the lid into place. Select Pressure Cook or Manual, and adjust the pressure to High and the time to 12 minutes. After cooking, let the pressure release naturally for 5 minutes, then quick release any remaining pressure.

4. Unlock the lid. Stir in the tomatoes and cilantro. Taste the beans and adjust the seasoning, if needed. If the beans are too soupy, select Sauté and adjust to Medium heat. Simmer until the beans thicken. Serve topped with the cheese and salsa.

Make It Vegetarian: Instead of the chorizo, use ¼ pound of chopped mushrooms. Heat 1 tablespoon extra-virgin olive oil to sauté the mushrooms, and add 1 minced garlic clove, ¼ teaspoon dried oregano, ½ teaspoon cumin, ¼ teaspoon smoked paprika, ½ teaspoon ancho chile powder, and a pinch ground cinnamon. Substitute vegetable stock for the chicken stock.

Use It Up: Use extra chorizo in the Chorizo and Green Chile Breakfast Casserole (page 32). Use the remaining Monterey Jack cheese in that casserole or the Creamy Salsa Verde Chicken (page 105), in which you can also use the extra salsa.

Southwestern Black Bean Salad

I based this recipe on a rice and vegetable salad I used to make years ago. I always thought the rice diluted the flavors of the salad, so I've upped the amount of beans and corn and left out the rice entirely. The result is a tangy, intensely flavored side dish that's perfect with grilled meats or Tex-Mex meals.

SERVES 2
AS A SIDE DISH

PREP & FINISHING:
10 MINUTES

PRESSURE COOK:
8 MINUTES HIGH

RELEASE:
NATURAL
10 MINUTES,
THEN QUICK

TOTAL TIME:
40 MINUTES,
PLUS 8 HOURS
TO SOAK

Per Serving
Calories: 280; Fat: 15 g;
Carbohydrates: 32 g;
Fiber: 7 g; Protein: 8 g;
Sodium: 312 mg

For the salad

2 ounces black beans

3 cups water, divided

2 teaspoons kosher salt, divided

½ cup frozen corn, thawed

¼ cup chopped red bell pepper

2 scallions, green part only, chopped

2 tablespoons chopped cilantro

For the dressing

2 tablespoons extra-virgin olive oil

1 tablespoon freshly squeezed lime juice

¼ teaspoon kosher salt

¼ teaspoon ground cumin

¼ teaspoon ancho chile powder

1. Place the beans in a small bowl. Add 2 cups of water and 1½ teaspoons of salt. Let soak at room temperature for 6 to 8 hours. Drain and rinse.

2. Place the soaked beans in the inner pot. Add the remaining 1 cup of water and ½ teaspoon of salt. Lock the lid into place. Select Pressure Cook or Manual, and adjust the pressure to High and the time to 8 minutes.

3. While the beans are cooking, chop the vegetables and prepare the dressing. To make the dressing, place all the ingredients in a small jar with a tight-fitting lid. Shake to combine. If you don't have a jar, whisk the ingredients in a small bowl.

4. After cooking, let the pressure release naturally for 10 minutes, then quick release any remaining pressure.

5. Unlock the lid. Drain the beans into a strainer or colander, then transfer to a medium bowl. Shake or whisk the dressing and pour it over the beans. Let them cool in the dressing for 10 minutes, then stir in the corn, bell pepper, scallions, and cilantro.

Double It: Double all the ingredients (cook for the same amount of time), add some chopped Perfect Chicken Breast (page 104) or cooked shrimp, and you have a satisfying lunch or dinner.

Brown Rice and Broccoli Cheese Casserole

This updated version of the 1960s casserole uses brown rice, fresh broccoli, and real Cheddar cheese instead of a can of cheese soup. It's versatile—it's delicious on its own, you can also add a Perfect Chicken Breast (page 104) for a more substantial main dish, or you can serve it as a side if you prefer.

4 ounces broccoli florets

½ teaspoon kosher salt, divided

¾ cup brown rice, rinsed

¾ cup low-sodium chicken or vegetable broth

2 scallions, chopped, green and white parts separated

1 cup grated sharp Cheddar cheese

2 tablespoons heavy (whipping) cream

1. Place the broccoli in a steamer basket. Add 1 cup of water to the inner pot and place the steamer basket inside. Lock the lid into place. Select Steam and adjust the pressure to High and the time to 0 minutes. After cooking, quick release the pressure. Remove the broccoli and sprinkle with ¼ teaspoon of salt. Set aside.

2. Empty the inner pot and return it to the base. Add the rice, broth, white scallion parts, and the remaining ¼ teaspoon of salt.

3. Lock the lid into place. Select Pressure Cook or Manual; set the heat to High and the time to 22 minutes.

4. While the rice cooks, chop the broccoli into small bite-size pieces.

5. After cooking, let the pressure release naturally for 10 minutes, then quick release any remaining pressure.

6. Unlock the lid. Add the cheese and cream. Stir to melt the cheese. Gently stir in the broccoli and scallion greens. Serve.

Time Saver: You can use frozen thawed broccoli instead of fresh broccoli. There's no need to cook it. Just drain thoroughly and add it in step 6 to warm through.

Use It Up: Use extra broccoli in the Cilantro-Coconut Shrimp and Broccoli (page 100).

SERVES 2
AS A MAIN COURSE

PREP & FINISHING:
5 MINUTES

SAUTÉ:
4 MINUTES

PRESSURE COOK:
0 MINUTES HIGH
THEN 22 MINUTES
HIGH

RELEASE:
QUICK *THEN*
NATURAL
10 MINUTES,
THEN QUICK

TOTAL TIME:
55 MINUTES

Per Serving
Calories: 567; Fat: 26 g;
Carbohydrates: 16 g;
Fiber: 4 g; Protein: 22 g;
Sodium: 394 mg

Greek Salad with Bulgur Wheat

This dish is my combination of Middle Eastern tabbouleh and Greek salad. It's got more bulgur than a traditional tabbouleh, but keeps the same bold use of parsley and mint. Cucumbers, tomatoes, olives, and feta cheese come from the Greek side of the table. Together, the flavors and textures make a great light lunch dish. Campari tomatoes are small hothouse-grown tomatoes. They have an intense tomato flavor year-round and the small size makes them ideal when you're cooking for two.

SERVES 2
AS A LIGHT
MAIN DISH

PREP & FINISHING:
10 MINUTES

PRESSURE COOK:
0 MINUTES HIGH

RELEASE:
NATURAL
2 MINUTES,
THEN QUICK

TOTAL TIME:
25 MINUTES

Per Serving
Calories: 352; Fat: 32 g;
Carbohydrates: 14 g;
Fiber: 3 g; Protein: 6 g;
Sodium: 328 mg

½ cup coarse bulgur wheat

½ cup water

¼ teaspoon kosher salt

⅓ cup chopped English cucumber

½ cup chopped fresh cherry tomatoes

1 scallion, green part only, sliced

2 tablespoons coarsely chopped Kalamata olives

¼ cup extra-virgin olive oil

2 tablespoons freshly squeezed lemon juice

⅓ cup crumbled feta cheese

1 tablespoon chopped fresh mint

¼ cup chopped fresh parsley

1. Pour the bulgur into the inner pot. Add the water and kosher salt. Lock the lid into place. Select Pressure Cook or Manual, and adjust the pressure to High and the time to 0 minutes. After cooking, let the pressure release naturally for 2 minutes, then quick release any remaining pressure.

2. Unlock the lid. Remove the pot from the base. Fluff the bulgur with a fork and let it cool for a few minutes. Transfer it to a medium bowl.

3. Add the cucumber, tomatoes, scallion, and olives, and toss to combine. Drizzle with the olive oil and lemon juice. Add the feta cheese, mint, and parsley, and toss gently. Adjust the seasoning, adding salt or pepper as needed.

Make It Gluten-Free: Substitute cooked quinoa for the bulgur (see directions in the Quinoa with Marinated Artichokes and Peppers on page 71).

Use It Up: Extra feta can go in the Lentils with Red Peppers and Feta (page 67).

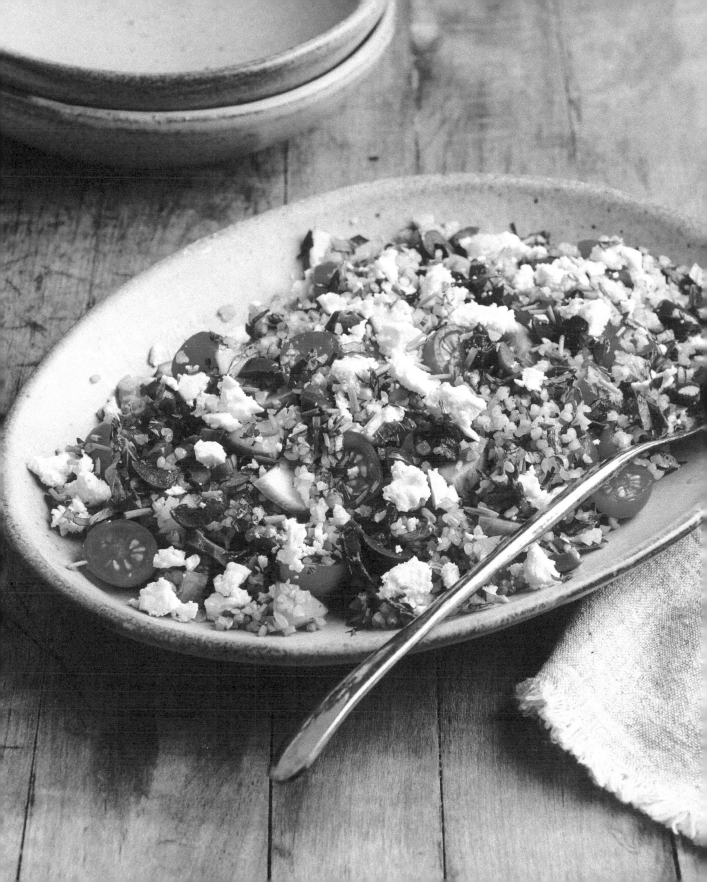

Rice Pilaf with Bacon and Water Chestnuts

This pilaf can be thought of as an Instant Pot® version of fried rice. The savory mixture of rice and vegetables makes a great side dish for any Asian-inspired meats, or you can add more bacon and a scrambled egg to make it a light lunch. If you don't have snow peas, you can add frozen thawed green peas instead.

SERVES 2 AS
A SIDE DISH

PREP & FINISHING:
10 MINUTES

SAUTÉ:
5 MINUTES

PRESSURE COOK:
0 MINUTES HIGH
THEN 8 MINUTES
HIGH

RELEASE:
QUICK *THEN*
QUICK

TOTAL TIME:
40 MINUTES

Per Serving
Calories: 303; Fat: 8 g;
Carbohydrates: 44 g;
Fiber: 2 g; Protein: 12 g;
Sodium: 724 mg

2 ounces snow peas
2 bacon slices, cut into
    ¼-inch-wide strips
¼ cup chopped onion
½ cup long-grain white rice

½ cup low-sodium chicken or
    vegetable stock
1 teaspoon soy sauce
½ cup chopped water chestnuts

1. Place the snow peas in a steamer basket. Add 1 cup of water to the inner pot and place the steamer basket inside. Lock the lid into place. Select Steam and adjust the pressure to High and the time to 0 minutes.

2. While the peas steam as the pot comes to pressure, chop the remaining vegetables.

3. After cooking, quick release the pressure.

4. Unlock the lid. Remove the trivet and peas and set aside. Empty the water from the pot and return it to the base.

5. Select Sauté and adjust to Medium heat. Add the bacon and cook, stirring occasionally, for about 4 minutes, or until the bacon is mostly crisp and the fat is rendered. Add the onion and cook, stirring often, until the onion pieces separate and soften. Add the rice and stir to coat in the fat, cooking for about 1 minute. Add the stock and soy sauce.

6. Lock the lid into place. Select Pressure Cook or Manual, and adjust the pressure to High and the time to 8 minutes. After cooking, quick release any remaining pressure.

7. Unlock the lid. Add the snow peas and water chestnuts. Stir gently to combine. Put the lid on the Instant Pot® but do not lock it into place. Let the pilaf sit for 5 to 6 minutes, or until the rice is completely cooked and the remaining ingredients are warmed through. Fluff with a fork and serve.

Make It A Meal: This dish is great with Char Siu (page 134) or Korean Short Ribs (page 122).

Use It Up: Use the other half of the water chestnuts in the Spicy Chicken Lettuce Cups (page 108). Use any remaining snow peas in the Spicy Sesame Noodles and Vegetables (page 85).

Herbed Wild Rice Pilaf with Almonds

The wild rice and brown rice combine to make a nutty, hearty pilaf. Wild rice—not a true rice, but a grass—pressure cooks at the same rate as brown rice, so they make a perfect pair. But you can also make this dish with all brown or all wild rice, if that's what you have on hand.

SERVES 2
AS A SIDE DISH

PREP & FINISHING:
5 MINUTES

SAUTÉ:
4 MINUTES

PRESSURE COOK:
22 MINUTES HIGH

RELEASE:
NATURAL
10 MINUTES,
THEN QUICK

TOTAL TIME:
50 MINUTES

Per Serving
Calories: 257; Fat: 17 g;
Carbohydrates: 22 g;
Fiber: 2 g; Protein: 5 g;
Sodium: 190 mg

2 tablespoons extra-virgin olive oil

1 tablespoon chopped onion or shallot

¼ cup wild rice

¼ cup long-grain brown rice, rinsed

½ cup low-sodium chicken or vegetable stock

1 bay leaf

1 fresh thyme sprig or ¼ teaspoon dried thyme

1 fresh oregano sprig or ¼ teaspoon dried oregano

½ teaspoon kosher salt

2 tablespoons toasted slivered almonds

2 tablespoons minced fresh parsley

1. Select Sauté and adjust to Medium heat. Add the olive oil and heat until shimmering. Add the onion and cook, stirring often, until the onion pieces separate and soften, about 2 minutes. Add the wild rice and brown rice and stir to coat, cooking for about 1 minute. Add the stock, bay leaf, thyme, oregano, and salt, and stir to combine.

2. Lock the lid into place. Select Pressure Cook or Manual, and adjust the pressure to High and the time to 22 minutes. After cooking, let the pressure release naturally for 10 minutes, then quick release any remaining pressure.

3. Unlock the lid. Fluff the rice with a fork and taste; if it's not quite done, just replace the lid (not locked) and let it steam for a few more minutes. Adjust the seasoning as necessary, and remove the bay leaf, thyme stem, and oregano stem. Just before serving, stir in the almonds and parsley.

Double It: For an easy main dish, double the recipe. Use double the ingredients (although just one of each herb sprig is fine) and the same cooking time. Stir in 4 to 6 ounces of Perfect Chicken Breast (page 104) along with the almonds and parsley.

Lentils with Red Peppers and Feta

I got the idea for this combination of ingredients from the delightful book Fresh & Fast Vegetarian *by Marie Simmons. I've streamlined it somewhat, using roasted peppers from a jar and cooking in the Instant Pot® to put the dish together even faster.*

2 tablespoons extra-virgin olive oil

½ small onion, chopped

2 garlic cloves, minced (about 2 teaspoons)

1 cup green or brown lentils, rinsed

2¼ cups low-sodium vegetable stock

½ teaspoon kosher salt

1 (7-ounce) jar roasted red peppers, drained and peppers patted dry

2 teaspoons freshly squeezed lemon juice

3 ounces feta cheese, crumbled

2 tablespoons chopped fresh parsley

SERVES 2
AS A MAIN DISH

PREP & FINISHING:
5 MINUTES

SAUTÉ:
4 MINUTES

PRESSURE COOK:
20 MINUTES HIGH

RELEASE:
NATURAL
10 MINUTES,
THEN QUICK

TOTAL TIME:
45 MINUTES

Per Serving
Calories: 647; Fat: 24 g;
Carbohydrates: 74 g;
Fiber: 32 g; Protein: 34 g;
Sodium: 623 mg

1. Select Sauté and adjust to Medium heat. Heat the olive oil until it shimmers. Add the onion and cook until soft, about 3 minutes. Add the garlic and cook until fragrant, about 1 minute. Add the lentils, stock, and salt.

2. Lock the lid in place. Select Pressure Cook or Manual, and adjust the pressure to High and the time to 20 minutes.

3. While the lentils are cooking, purée the peppers and lemon juice using an immersion blender (or mince the peppers and stir in the lemon juice).

4. After cooking, let the pressure release naturally for 10 minutes, then quick release any remaining pressure.

5. Unlock the lid. Stir the lentils and add the red pepper purée. Stir gently and let sit for a few minutes, until the purée warms. Serve topped with the feta and parsley.

Use It Up: Extra feta cheese can be used for the Greek Salad with Bulgur Wheat (page 62).

Jamaican Rice and Peas

In Jamaica, the "peas" in rice and peas are actually beans. Usually, red kidney beans are used, but I don't much like them, so I use small red beans instead. Cooked in coconut milk and spices, the rice and beans are creamy and flavorful. The chile doesn't add much heat since it's left whole, but it does give some flavor and a hint of spice.

SERVES 2 AS
A SIDE DISH

PREP & FINISHING:
10 MINUTES

PRESSURE COOK:
8 MINUTES HIGH
THEN 4 MINUTES
HIGH

RELEASE:
NATURAL
5 MINUTES,
THEN QUICK *THEN*
NATURAL
10 MINUTES,
THEN QUICK

TOTAL TIME:
55 MINUTES, PLUS
8 HOURS TO SOAK

Per Serving
Calories: 727; Fat: 48 g;
Carbohydrates: 67 g;
Fiber: 10 g; Protein: 15 g;
Sodium: 365 mg

2 cups water

2½ teaspoons kosher
   salt, divided

2 ounces dried small red beans
   or kidney beans

1 (14-ounce) can coconut milk

1 garlic clove, lightly smashed

1 or 2 fresh ginger slices

¼ teaspoon ground allspice

¼ teaspoon freshly ground
   black pepper

2 fresh thyme sprigs

1 scallion, root trimmed

1 fresh Scotch bonnet or
   habanero chile (optional)

½ cup long-grain rice, rinsed

1. In a large bowl, add the water. Dissolve 1½ teaspoons of kosher salt in the water. Add the beans and soak at room temperature for 8 to 24 hours. Drain and rinse.

2. Place the beans in the inner pot. Measure out 1 cup of coconut milk, reserving most of the fat, and pour the cup into the pot. Add the garlic, ginger, allspice, pepper, thyme, and ½ teaspoon of salt.

3. Lock the lid into place. Select Pressure Cook or Manual, and adjust the pressure to High and the time to 8 minutes. After cooking, let the pressure release naturally for 5 minutes, then quick release any remaining pressure.

4. Unlock the lid. Add the scallion and chile (if using). Pour in the rice and add 6 tablespoons of the remaining coconut milk (still reserving the fat) and the remaining ½ teaspoon of salt. Push the rice down into the liquid so it is fully submerged.

5. Lock the lid into place. Select Pressure Cook or Manual, and adjust the pressure to High and the time to 4 minutes. After cooking, let the pressure release naturally for 10 minutes, then quick release any remaining pressure.

6. Unlock the lid. Remove the garlic clove, ginger slices, scallion, and chile. Stir in a tablespoon or so of the fat from the coconut milk. Taste and adjust the seasonings, if needed.

Time Saver: You can use your own cooked or canned kidney beans (rinsed and drained) instead of cooking them here. Mix the rice with the aromatics in the inner pot and pour in ½ cup of the coconut milk liquid. Spoon the beans on top and cook for 4 minutes on High, with 10 minutes natural release. Remove the aromatics, and stir in the coconut fat.

Creamy Mushroom-Barley Soup

This hearty vegetarian soup is a delicious alternative to the more common beef and barley soup. It makes a great lunch or, with some bread and a salad, an easy dinner. Be sure to buy pearled barley, which will cook faster than hulled barley.

SERVES 2

PREP & FINISHING:
10 MINUTES

SAUTÉ:
4 MINUTES

PRESSURE COOK:
20 MINUTES HIGH

RELEASE:
NATURAL
10 MINUTES,
THEN QUICK

TOTAL TIME:
55 MINUTES

Per Serving
Calories: 532; Fat: 30 g;
Carbohydrates: 57 g;
Fiber: 11 g; Protein: 12 g;
Sodium: 242 mg

1 tablespoon extra-virgin olive oil
1 small onion, chopped
1 garlic clove, minced
1 carrot, cut into
   ½-inch-thick rounds
1 celery rib, sliced ¼ inch thick
½ cup pearled barley
8 ounces white button or cremini
   mushrooms, sliced
2 cups low-sodium
   vegetable broth

1 bay leaf
1 teaspoon dried thyme
¼ teaspoon kosher salt
¼ teaspoon freshly ground
   black pepper
½ teaspoon
   Worcestershire sauce
½ cup heavy (whipping) cream,
   or more as needed

1. Select Sauté and adjust to Medium heat. Add the olive oil and heat until it shimmers. Add the onion and garlic and cook, stirring often, until the onion pieces separate and soften. Add the carrot, celery, barley, mushrooms, broth, bay leaf, thyme, salt, and pepper to the pot.

2. Lock the lid into place. Select Pressure Cook or Manual, and adjust the pressure to High and the time to 20 minutes. After cooking, let the pressure release naturally for 10 minutes, then quick release any remaining pressure.

3. Unlock the lid. Stir in the Worcestershire sauce and cream to the soup. Let warm through.

Double It: The soup freezes well, so you can double it and freeze half. If you do freeze it, leave the cream out until you thaw and reheat it.

Make It Dairy-Free: The soup is also delicious without the cream, so you can just leave it out. Increase the olive oil to 2 tablespoons.

Quinoa with Marinated Artichokes and Peppers

Back when almost nobody had heard of quinoa, I was introduced to it in a salad with marinated vegetables and a light dressing. It's still the way I most enjoy quinoa, and this combination is one of my favorites.

¼ cup extra-virgin olive oil

2 tablespoons red or white wine vinegar

1 teaspoon minced garlic

¾ teaspoon kosher salt, divided

¼ teaspoon freshly ground black pepper

½ cup artichoke hearts (drained if canned, thawed if frozen)

¼ cup roasted red pepper, cut into strips

1 small shallot, thinly sliced

½ cup quinoa, rinsed

¾ cup water

2 tablespoons minced fresh parsley

1. Pour the olive oil into a medium bowl. Add the vinegar, garlic, ¼ teaspoon of salt, and the pepper. Whisk to combine. Add the artichoke hearts, roasted red peppers, and shallot, and stir to coat. Set aside.

2. Pour the rinsed quinoa into the inner pot. Add the water and the remaining ½ teaspoon of salt. Lock the lid into place. Select Pressure Cook or Manual, and adjust the pressure to High and the time to 1 minute. After cooking, let the pressure release naturally for 12 minutes, then quick release any remaining pressure.

3. Unlock the lid. Remove the pot from the base. Fluff the quinoa with a fork and let it cool for a few minutes. Spoon the quinoa into the bowl with the vegetables. Add the parsley and toss gently to coat the quinoa with the dressing.

Double It: Double all the ingredients—including the water for the quinoa—for a delicious and portable lunch.

Use It Up: Use leftover roasted red pepper in the Pimiento Cheese Corn Pudding (page 43).

SERVES 2 AS A SIDE DISH

PREP & FINISHING:
10 MINUTES

PRESSURE COOK:
1 MINUTE HIGH

RELEASE:
NATURAL 12 MINUTES, THEN QUICK

TOTAL TIME:
30 MINUTES

Per Serving
Calories: 407; Fat: 28 g; Carbohydrates: 34 g; Fiber: 6 g; Protein: 8 g; Sodium: 327 mg

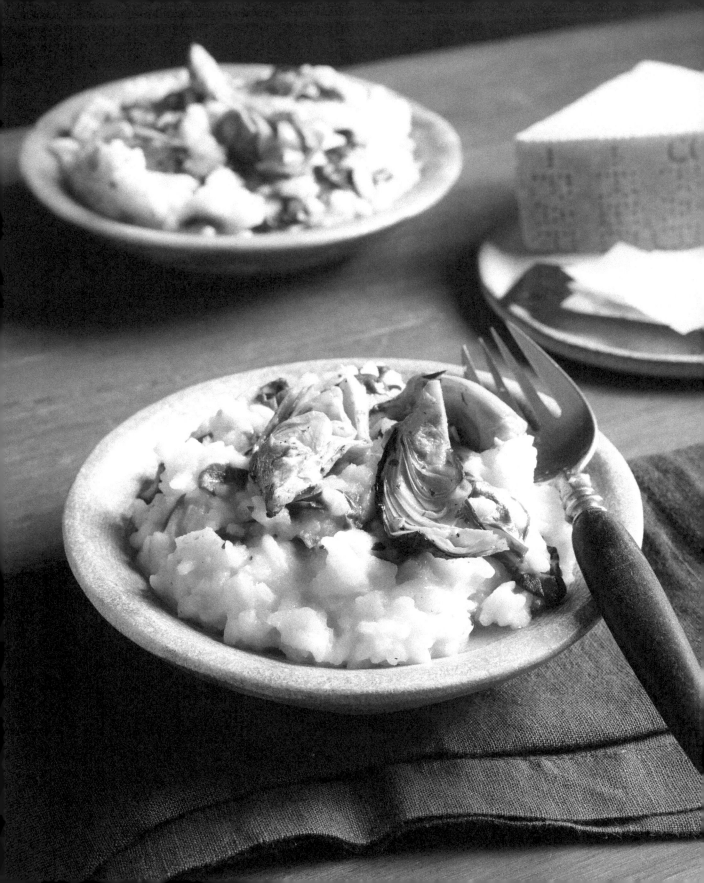

chapter 5
Meatless Mains

Minestrone . . . 74

Curried Cauliflower Soup . . . 76

Spaghetti Squash with Browned Butter and Parmesan . . . 77

Polenta with Mushroom Sauce . . . 78

Spicy Braised Tofu and Carrots . . . 80

Rotini with Creamy Basil and Sun-Dried Tomato Sauce . . . 81

Artichoke and Spinach Risotto . . . 82

Mushroom Stroganoff . . . 83

Spicy Sesame Noodles and Vegetables . . . 85

Vegetable Korma . . . 86

Artichoke and Spinach Risotto, page 82

Minestrone

Minestrone, or Italian vegetable soup, is an easy weeknight dinner. After a quick sauté, everything goes in the pot at once, and cooks for only a few minutes. Make some garlic bread while the soup cooks, and you're all set. If you buy Parmigiano or similar Parmesan cheeses, you can keep the rinds in the freezer for soups like this. It's not necessary, but it does add a lot of flavor.

SERVES 2

PREP & FINISHING:
10 MINUTES

SAUTÉ:
5 MINUTES

PRESSURE COOK:
5 MINUTES HIGH

RELEASE:
NATURAL
2 MINUTES,
THEN QUICK

TOTAL TIME:
30 MINUTES

Per Serving
Calories: 613; Fat: 26 g;
Carbohydrates: 76 g;
Fiber: 19 g; Protein: 25 g;
Sodium: 821 mg

3 tablespoons extra-virgin olive oil
½ small onion, diced
1 small carrot, diced
1 teaspoon minced garlic
½ zucchini, diced
½ (14-ounce) can diced tomatoes
1 (15-ounce) can cannellini beans, drained and rinsed
1½ cups low-sodium vegetable stock

2 ounces elbow macaroni (about ½ cup)
1 bay leaf
1 teaspoon Italian dried herbs, or ½ teaspoon dried oregano and ½ teaspoon dried basil
¼ teaspoon red pepper flakes
½ teaspoon kosher salt
1 Parmesan rind (optional)
2 cups baby spinach
¼ cup grated Parmesan cheese
3 tablespoons pesto (optional)

1. Select Sauté and adjust to Medium heat. Pour the olive oil into the inner pot and heat until shimmering. Add the onion, carrot, and garlic and cook, stirring occasionally, about 5 minutes, or until the vegetables start to soften. Add the zucchini, tomatoes, beans, stock, macaroni, bay leaf, Italian herbs, red pepper flakes, salt, and Parmesan rind (if using).

2. Lock the lid into place. Select Pressure Cook or Manual, and adjust the pressure to High and the time to 5 minutes. After cooking, let the pressure release naturally for 2 minutes, then quick release any remaining pressure.

3. Unlock the lid. Remove and discard the Parmesan rind and bay leaf. Stir in the spinach. When it's wilted, serve the soup topped with the grated Parmesan cheese and pesto (if using).

Double It: Double all the ingredients, but reduce the cooking time by 1 minute.

Mini Modification: In step 2, cook for 4 minutes instead of 5 minutes.

Use It Up: Use the other half of the zucchini in Thai Red Curry Beef (page 129). Use the other half of the tomatoes in Easy Chili (page 123) or Vegetable Korma (page 86).

Curried Cauliflower Soup

This cauliflower soup gets a boost of flavor from browning the cauliflower before pressure cooking. The curry flavor, accented with a hint of orange, is mild—use more if you like a pronounced curry flavor. I like this soup with a drizzle of cream to finish, but it's just as delicious without it.

SERVES 2 AS A
MAIN COURSE

PREP & FINISHING:
10 MINUTES

SAUTÉ:
5 MINUTES

PRESSURE COOK:
3 MINUTES HIGH

RELEASE:
NATURAL
10 MINUTES,
THEN QUICK

TOTAL TIME:
40 MINUTES

Per Serving
Calories: 257; Fat: 15 g;
Carbohydrates: 30 g;
Fiber: 8 g; Protein: 6 g;
Sodium: 349 mg

2 tablespoons extra-virgin olive oil

3 cups cauliflower florets (about 1 pound trimmed, or ½ a large head), divided

1 small (about 6 ounces) russet potato, peeled and cut into 1-inch chunks

1 medium onion, chopped

2 garlic cloves

2 teaspoons curry powder (or more as needed)

¼ teaspoon orange juice concentrate (optional)

1 teaspoon kosher salt

2 cups water

1 tablespoon heavy (whipping) cream (optional)

2 tablespoons minced fresh chives

1. Select Sauté and adjust to Medium heat. Add the olive oil to the inner pot and heat until shimmering. Add about 1 cup of cauliflower florets (just enough to cover the bottom of the pot) and let brown, without stirring or turning, for about 3 minutes, or until the florets are browned on one side. Turn over the florets and brown for another 2 minutes, without stirring, on the other side.

2. Add the remaining 2 cups of cauliflower, potato, onion, garlic, curry powder, orange juice concentrate (if using), salt, and water.

3. Lock the lid into place. Select Pressure Cook or Manual, and adjust the pressure to High and the time to 3 minutes. After cooking, let the pressure release naturally for 10 minutes, then quick release any remaining pressure lid.

4. Unlock the lid. Using an immersion blender (or stand blender), purée the soup. Adjust the seasoning, adding more salt or curry powder as desired. Garnish by drizzling the cream over the top (if using). Sprinkle with chives and serve.

Make It Dairy-Free: Omit the cream garnish, substituting extra-virgin olive oil, if desired.

Use It Up: Use any extra cauliflower in the Vegetable Korma (page 86).

Spaghetti Squash with Browned Butter and Parmesan

When I was in high school, I loved going to the Old Spaghetti Factory in Seattle, and I especially loved spaghetti with browned butter and mizithra cheese. I've based this recipe for spaghetti squash on my old favorite, but I use Parmesan cheese because it's easier to find.

1 small (2- to 3-pound) spaghetti squash

4 tablespoons unsalted butter

¼ teaspoon kosher salt

⅛ teaspoon freshly ground black pepper

½ cup grated Parmesan cheese, divided

2 tablespoons chopped parsley (optional)

SERVES 2

PREP & FINISHING:
10 MINUTES

PRESSURE COOK:
7 MINUTES HIGH

RELEASE:
QUICK

SAUTÉ:
4 MINUTES

TOTAL TIME:
30 MINUTES

Per Serving
Calories: 435; Fat: 32 g; Carbohydrates: 32 g; Fiber: 1 g; Protein: 12 g; Sodium: 379 mg

1. Cut the squash in half lengthwise and scoop out the seeds.

2. Pour 1 cup of water into the inner pot and place the trivet inside. Place the squash halves on the trivet, cut-side down if possible. Lock the lid into place. Select Steam and adjust the pressure to High and the time to 7 minutes. After cooking, quick release the pressure.

3. Unlock the lid. Remove the squash halves and the trivet. Set the squash aside to cool for a couple of minutes.

4. Empty the inner pot, dry it, and return it to the base. Select Sauté and adjust to Medium heat. Add the butter. After it melts, continue to cook until the milk solids begin to brown, about 4 minutes.

5. While the butter browns, scrape out the squash flesh with a fork to form long strands. Place the squash in a colander to drain for a few minutes, then transfer to a medium bowl.

6. When the butter is browned, drizzle it over the squash. Sprinkle each half with the salt, pepper, and ¼ cup of Parmesan cheese. Toss gently. Spoon onto two plates and top each with the remaining ¼ cup of Parmesan and the parsley (if using).

Easier Together: One cook can tend to shredding and draining the squash, while the other browns the butter, grates the cheese, and chops the parsley.

Polenta with Mushroom Sauce

Garlic, red pepper flakes, and fennel seed give this hearty mushroom sauce the flavors of Italian sausage. Served over cheese-enriched polenta, it makes an elegant and delicious meatless dinner for two. A green salad is a great accompaniment.

SERVES 2

PREP & FINISHING:
10 MINUTES

SAUTÉ:
7 MINUTES

PRESSURE COOK:
15 MINUTES HIGH

RELEASE:
NATURAL
10 MINUTES,
THEN QUICK

TOTAL TIME:
50 MINUTES

Per Serving
Calories: 565; Fat: 30 g;
Carbohydrates: 53 g;
Fiber: 7 g; Protein: 18 g;
Sodium: 407 mg

2 tablespoons extra-virgin olive oil

½ small onion, sliced

2 garlic cloves, minced (about 2 teaspoons)

½ cup white wine

1 pound mushrooms (any mixture), sliced

1 (14-ounce) can diced tomatoes

1 teaspoon kosher salt, divided

¼ teaspoon red pepper flakes

¼ teaspoon fennel seeds

½ cup polenta or grits (not instant or quick-cook)

1 cup whole milk

1 cup low-sodium vegetable stock or Mushroom Stock (page 159)

2 tablespoons unsalted butter

¼ cup grated Parmesan or similar cheese, plus more for finishing

1. Select Sauté and adjust to Medium heat. Add the olive oil to the inner pot and heat until shimmering. Add the onion and cook until soft, about 3 minutes. Add the garlic and cook until fragrant, about 1 minute. Pour in the wine and let simmer for about 3 minutes, or until it is reduced by about half.

2. Add the mushrooms, tomatoes with their juice, ½ teaspoon of salt, red pepper flakes, and fennel seeds. Stir to combine. Place a trivet in the pot that's tall enough to clear the mushroom mixture.

3. In a heat-proof bowl that holds at least 4 cups, add the polenta. Add the milk, stock, and remaining ½ teaspoon of salt. Stir. Place the bowl on the trivet.

4. Lock the lid into place. Select Manual, and adjust the pressure to High and the time to 15 minutes. After cooking, let the pressure release naturally for 10 minutes, then quick release any remaining pressure.

5. Unlock the lid. Carefully remove the bowl of polenta. Stir the polenta until it's smooth (it may be clumpy at first). Add the butter and Parmesan cheese to the polenta and stir again to melt the butter and cheese. Taste and adjust the seasoning as necessary. Set aside.

6. Stir the mushroom sauce and taste for seasoning. If it's too thin, select Sauté and adjust to Medium heat. Simmer until the sauce has thickened.

7. To serve, spoon the polenta into bowls and top with the mushroom sauce. Sprinkle with additional cheese, if desired.

Double It: The mushroom sauce can be doubled (the extra freezes well). The cooking time remains the same.

Easier Together: One of you can start the sauce while the other person slices the mushrooms.

Spicy Braised Tofu and Carrots

Inspired by the Korean banchan dish dubu-jorim, *this braised tofu dish makes a great vegetarian entrée by itself or served with rice. I like carrots in the dish since they cook at the same quick rate as the tofu, but you could also stir in baby spinach after cooking, stirring to wilt it.*

8 ounces firm tofu, cut into
    1-inch cubes
2 medium carrots, cut into
    1-inch chunks
1 tablespoon soy sauce
1 tablespoon sugar
1 scallion, thinly sliced, green and
    white parts separated

2 garlic cloves, minced
1 teaspoon red pepper flakes
⅓ cup water
1 tablespoon sesame oil
1 teaspoon toasted
    sesame seeds

SERVES 2

PREP & FINISHING:
10 MINUTES

PRESSURE COOK:
4 MINUTES HIGH

RELEASE:
QUICK

TOTAL TIME:
25 MINUTES

Per Serving
Calories: 210; Fat: 13 g;
Carbohydrates: 17 g;
Fiber: 3 g; Protein: 11 g;
Sodium: 509 mg

1. Place the tofu and carrots in the inner pot. Add the soy sauce, sugar, white scallion parts, garlic, red pepper flakes, and water.

2. Lock the lid into place. Select Pressure Cook or Manual, and adjust the pressure to High and the time to 4 minutes. After cooking, quick release the pressure.

3. Unlock the lid. Stir in the sesame oil, and adjust the seasonings as necessary. If you like, simmer for 2 to 3 minutes to thicken the sauce. Serve garnished with the sesame seeds and scallion greens.

Make It Gluten-Free: Substitute gluten-free tamari for the soy sauce.

Mini Modification: Cook for 3 minutes.

Rotini with Creamy Basil
and Sun-Dried Tomato Sauce

There's something so comforting about pasta with a creamy tomato sauce. This one is extra flavorful, made with sun-dried tomato paste, which you can find in your local market (I find it in the produce section). If you can't find the sun-dried paste, you can make your own from a jar of sun-dried tomatoes packed in oil, puréeing it with an immersion blender.

5 ounces rotini pasta

1 teaspoon extra-virgin olive oil

½ teaspoon kosher salt

¼ teaspoon red pepper flakes

2 garlic cloves, minced (about 2 teaspoons)

1¼ cups water

¼ cup sun-dried tomato paste

½ cup heavy (whipping) cream

1 cup cherry tomatoes, halved

⅓ cup grated Parmesan cheese, plus additional to garnish

¼ cup chopped fresh basil, plus additional to garnish

SERVES 2

PREP & FINISHING:
10 MINUTES

SAUTÉ:
3 MINUTES

PRESSURE COOK:
5 MINUTES HIGH

RELEASE:
QUICK

TOTAL TIME:
30 MINUTES

Per Serving
Calories: 668; Fat: 36 g;
Carbohydrates: 62 g;
Fiber: 4 g; Protein: 19 g;
Sodium: 765 mg

1. Place the pasta in the inner pot. Add the olive oil, salt, red pepper flakes, garlic, water, and sun-dried tomato paste. Stir to combine.

2. Lock the lid into place. Select Pressure Cook or Manual, and adjust the pressure to High and the time to 5 minutes. After cooking, quick release the pressure.

3. Unlock the lid. Stir the cream and tomatoes into the pasta. Select Sauté and adjust to Medium heat. Bring the cream to a simmer and cook until thickened slightly, about 3 minutes. Gently stir in the cheese and basil. Serve with more cheese or basil, if desired.

Double It: If you have a 6-quart Instant Pot®, you can double the recipe. Double all the ingredients, and cook for 4 minutes. It's not recommended doubling the recipe in the Mini.

Use It Up: Use extra sun-dried tomatoes purée in the Marinara Sauce (page 160). Use extra basil in the Warm Thai-Style Green Bean and Tomato Salad (page 50), the Thai Red Curry Beef (page 129), or the Italian Tuna and Bean Salad (page 102).

Artichoke and Spinach Risotto

When I was first introduced to pressure cookers, risotto was one of the dishes that convinced me to buy one. I was skeptical that decent risotto was even possible without constant stirring, but amazingly, it is! I love the combination of artichokes and spinach in risotto, but try any cooked vegetables you like.

SERVES 2

PREP & FINISHING:
10 MINUTES

SAUTÉ:
6 MINUTES
THEN 3 MINUTES

PRESSURE COOK:
8 MINUTES HIGH

RELEASE:
QUICK

TOTAL TIME:
35 MINUTES

Per Serving
Calories: 287; Fat: 15 g;
Carbohydrates: 26 g;
Fiber: 5 g; Protein: 10 g;
Sodium: 502 mg

2 tablespoons unsalted butter, divided

½ small onion, chopped (about ¼ cup)

½ cup plus 2 tablespoons arborio rice

½ cup artichoke hearts (drained if canned, thawed if frozen)

¼ cup white wine

2 cups low-sodium vegetable stock, divided, plus more if needed

¼ teaspoon kosher salt

2 cups baby spinach

¼ cup grated Parmesan or similar cheese

1. Select Sauté and adjust to Medium heat. Add 1 tablespoon of butter to the inner pot. When it has stopped foaming, add the onion and cook, stirring, until the onion pieces separate and soften, about 3 minutes. Add the rice and stir to coat in the butter, cooking for about 1 minute. Stir in the artichoke hearts. Add the wine and cook, stirring, for 2 to 3 minutes, until it is almost evaporated.

2. Add 1¾ cups of stock and the salt, and stir to combine. Lock the lid into place. Select Pressure Cook or Manual, and adjust the pressure to High and the time to 8 minutes. After cooking, quick release the pressure.

3. Unlock the lid. Test the risotto; the rice should be soft with a slightly firm center and the sauce should be creamy, but it will probably not be quite done. Add another ¼ cup of stock and stir in the spinach. Select Sauté and adjust to Medium heat. Simmer for 2 to 3 minutes until the spinach is wilted and the sauce is creamy. If the rice is too dry, add more stock to loosen it up. Stir in the remaining 1 tablespoon of butter and the cheese. Taste and adjust the seasoning. Serve.

Use It Up: Extra spinach can go in the Congee with Eggs and Spinach (page 25) or Minestrone (page 74). Use the rest of your arborio rice in the Congee as well. The remaining artichokes can go in the Quinoa with Marinated Artichokes and Peppers (page 71).

Mushroom Stroganoff

When I was growing up, beef stroganoff was one of my mother's "company dishes." This version, made with all mushrooms instead of beef, is quicker to make and just as delicious. It's still fancy enough for company, too, if you double it.

1 tablespoon unsalted butter

½ small onion, thinly sliced

1 pound mushrooms (any mixture), sliced

½ cup dry sherry or white wine

2¼ cups Mushroom Stock (page 159)

1 teaspoon kosher salt

4 ounces egg noodles

¼ cup sour cream

2 tablespoons chopped fresh parsley, for garnish

SERVES 2

PREP & FINISHING:
10 MINUTES

SAUTÉ:
10 MINUTES

PRESSURE COOK:
5 MINUTES HIGH

RELEASE:
QUICK

TOTAL TIME:
35 MINUTES

Per Serving
Calories: 464; Fat: 15 g;
Carbohydrates: 58 g;
Fiber: 6 g; Protein: 18 g;
Sodium: 540 mg

1. Select Sauté and adjust to Medium heat. Add the butter to the inner pot and heat until it foams. Add the onion and cook, stirring occasionally, for about 3 minutes, or until the onion pieces start to soften. Add the mushrooms and cook, stirring occasionally, until they begin to soften, about 3 minutes. Pour in the sherry and bring to a simmer. Cook for 2 to 3 minutes to cook off some of the alcohol and let the liquid reduce by about half. Add the stock, salt, and noodles. Stir to combine.

2. Lock the lid into place. Select Pressure Cook or Manual, and adjust the pressure to High and the time to 5 minutes. After cooking, quick release the pressure.

3. Unlock the lid. Let the mushrooms and noodles rest for a minute or so, until the sauce is barely simmering and cools slightly before adding the sour cream. Stir in the sour cream. Ladle into bowls and garnish with the parsley.

Double It: Double all the ingredients, but reduce the cooking time to 4 minutes.

Mini Modification: Reduce the cooking time to 4 minutes.

Use It Up: Use extra egg noodles in the Chicken Paprikash (page 112).

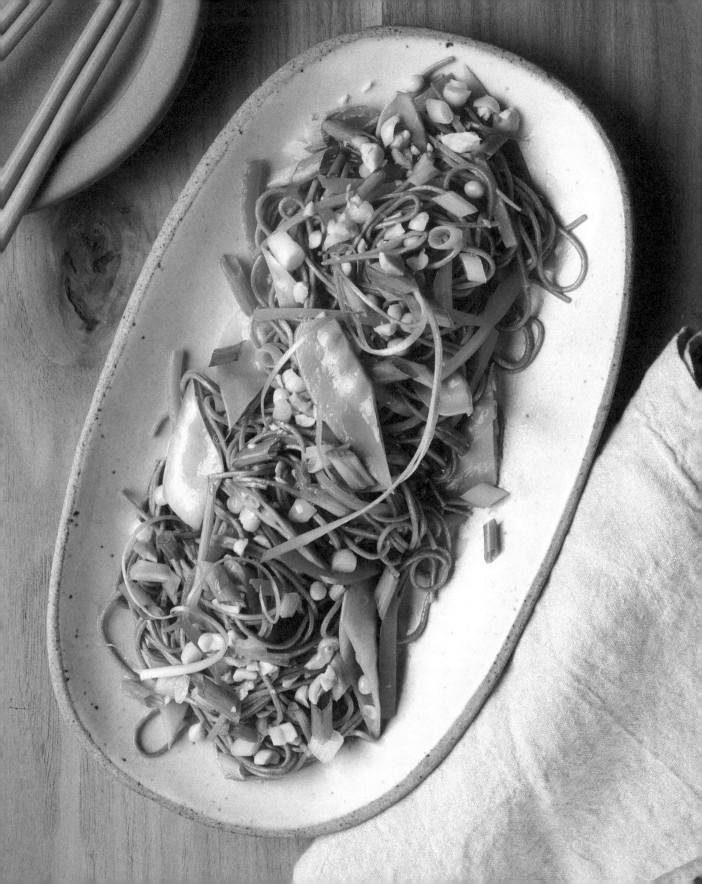

Spicy Sesame Noodles and Vegetables

When I discovered I could cook Chinese noodles in the Instant Pot®, my life changed. Okay, not really—but it was a great trick to have up my sleeve. For noodles, I use the KA-ME brand, but you can also substitute ramen noodles. In this recipe, the noodles cook at the same rate as the vegetables, and the cooking liquid turns into a sauce. Dinner is served!

1¼ cups water

1 tablespoon soy sauce

2 tablespoons sesame oil, divided

1 garlic clove, minced

1 tablespoon Asian chili-garlic sauce or Sriracha, plus additional as needed

4 ounces Chinese wheat noodles or 1 (4-ounce) package ramen noodles

3 ounces snow peas, trimmed (about 1 cup)

1 small carrot, cut into thin matchsticks

1 small red bell pepper, cut into thin strips

2 or 3 scallions, chopped, green and white parts separated

2 tablespoons coarsely chopped roasted peanuts (optional)

SERVES 2

PREP & FINISHING:
10 MINUTES

PRESSURE COOK:
0 MINUTES LOW

RELEASE:
QUICK

TOTAL TIME:
25 MINUTES

Per Serving
Calories: 456; Fat: 15 g;
Carbohydrates: 69 g;
Fiber: 9 g; Protein: 17 g;
Sodium: 542 mg

1. Add the water to the inner pot. Add the soy sauce, 1 tablespoon of sesame oil, the garlic, and chili-garlic sauce. Stir to combine. Break up the block of noodles into 3 or 4 pieces and place them in the pot in a single layer as much as possible. Layer the snow peas, carrot, bell pepper, and white scallion parts over the noodles.

2. Lock the lid into place. Select Pressure Cook or Manual, and adjust the pressure to Low and the time to 0 minutes. After cooking, quick release the pressure.

3. Unlock the lid. Stir the noodles and vegetables together. Test a noodle and a carrot to make sure both are tender. If not, simmer for a few minutes until they're done. Stir in the remaining 1 tablespoon of sesame oil and more chili-garlic sauce if you'd like. Garnish with the scallion greens and peanuts (if using).

Use It Up: Use the remaining noodles in the Cilantro-Coconut Shrimp and Broccoli (page 100). If you have leftover snow peas, use them in the Rice Pilaf with Bacon and Water Chestnuts (page 64).

Lux Modification: In step 1, use hot water rather than room temperature; keep the time the same.

Vegetable Korma

One of the best Indian dishes I've ever had was a really spicy vegetable korma from a takeout place in San Francisco. This dish is a pretty good homage, if I do say so myself. It certainly satisfies those cravings, and I don't have to wait for delivery.

SERVES 2

PREP & FINISHING:
10 MINUTES

PRESSURE COOK:
2 MINUTES HIGH
THEN 2 MINUTES
LOW

RELEASE:
QUICK *THEN*
QUICK

TOTAL TIME:
30 MINUTES

Per Serving
Calories: 316; Fat: 17 g;
Carbohydrates: 38 g;
Fiber: 9 g; Protein: 8 g;
Sodium: 333 mg

½ (14-ounce) can diced tomatoes, drained
½ cup coconut milk
½ small onion, chopped
1 jalapeño, seeded and sliced
3 garlic cloves, smashed
1 teaspoon garam masala
½ teaspoon kosher salt
½ teaspoon ground turmeric
¼ teaspoon cumin
½ teaspoon red pepper flakes, plus more as needed

1 tablespoon cashew or almond butter (optional)
1 small (6- to 8-ounce) russet potato, peeled and cut into 1-inch cubes
1 medium carrot, cut into 1-inch chunks
1 cup cauliflower florets
½ cup frozen green peas
¼ cup chopped cilantro, for garnish
¼ cup roasted unsalted cashews or almonds, for garnish

1. Add the tomatoes and coconut milk to the inner pot. Add the onion, jalapeño, garlic, garam masala, salt, turmeric, cumin, red pepper flakes, and nut butter (if using).

2. Place the potato and carrot chunks into a steamer basket. Place the basket in the inner pot on top of the sauce ingredients. Lock the lid into place. Select Pressure Cook or Manual, and adjust the pressure to High and the time to 2 minutes. After cooking, quick release the pressure. Unlock the lid. Remove the steamer basket and set aside.

3. Using an immersion blender, purée the sauce until smooth. Adjust the seasoning, if necessary. Transfer the potatoes and carrots into the inner pot. Add the cauliflower and peas and stir to coat the vegetables with the sauce.

4. Lock the lid into place. Select Pressure Cook or Manual, and adjust the pressure to Low and the time to 2 minutes. After cooking, quick release the pressure. Unlock the lid. Stir and adjust the seasoning, if necessary.

5. Serve the korma over Basic White or Brown Rice (page 163), if you like, and garnish with the cilantro and cashews.

Lux Modification: Use high pressure for the second cooking in step 4 and keep the time the same.

Make It Nut-Free: The nut butter is there mostly to thicken the sauce, so if you have a nut allergy, just leave it out and omit the nut garnish.

Use It Up: Use the other half of the can of tomatoes in the Minestrone (page 74) or Easy Chili (page 123). Use extra cauliflower in the Curried Cauliflower Soup (page 76).

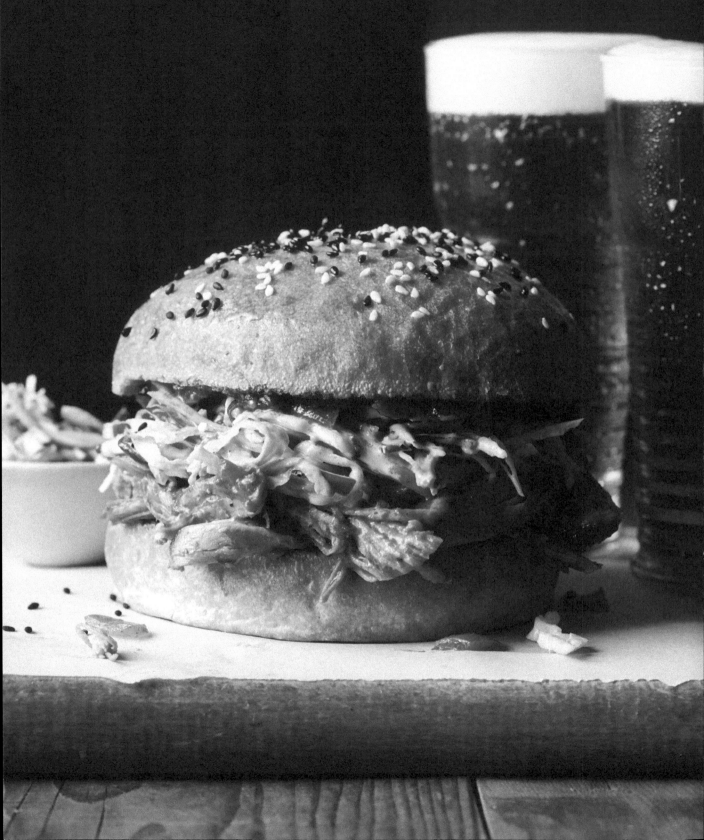

chapter 6
Seafood and Poultry

Scalloped Potatoes with Smoked Salmon . . . 90

Farfalle with Salmon, Fennel, and Tomatoes . . . 92

Cod and Green Beans with Dill Mustard Sauce . . . 94

Clam Chowder . . . 96

Shrimp and Grits . . . 98

Cilantro-Coconut Shrimp and Broccoli . . . 100

Italian Tuna and Bean Salad . . . 102

Perfect Chicken Breast . . . 104

Creamy Salsa Verde Chicken . . . 105

Shawarma-Style Chicken and Rice . . . 106

Spicy Chicken Lettuce Cups . . . 108

Chicken Thighs with Salami and Fennel . . . 110

Chicken Paprikash . . . 112

Teriyaki Chicken and Rice . . . 113

Sweet and Sour Chicken . . . 114

Chicken Noodle Soup . . . 115

Barbecue Chicken Sandwiches with Slaw . . . 116

Turkey and Stuffing for Two . . . 118

Barbecue Chicken Sandwiches with Slaw, page 116

Scalloped Potatoes with Smoked Salmon

In Sweden, this traditional comfort food is called Lax Pudding (my guess is that "lax" is short for "gravlax")—an odd name, to American ears, for a delicious dish. The result is like scalloped potatoes and smoked salmon, with just enough custard to hold it together. It's a great for brunch, paired with a tossed green salad or the Tangy Carrot and Celery Salad (page 45). You can use either hot-smoked salmon or cold-smoked lox (gravlax)—both are delicious.

SERVES 2

PREP & FINISHING:
15 MINUTES

PRESSURE COOK:
4 MINUTES HIGH
THEN 15 MINUTES
HIGH

RELEASE:
QUICK *THEN*
10 MINUTES
NATURAL,
THEN QUICK

TOTAL TIME:
55 MINUTES

Per Serving
Calories: 564; Fat: 39 g;
Carbohydrates: 28 g;
Fiber: 4 g; Protein: 28 g;
Sodium: 842 mg

9 ounces Yukon Gold potatoes (3 medium potatoes), peeled and cut into ¼-inch slices
¾ teaspoon kosher salt, divided
2 large eggs
½ cup whole milk
½ cup heavy (whipping) cream
¼ teaspoon freshly ground black pepper, plus more as needed
1 tablespoon unsalted butter, melted, divided
4 to 6 ounces smoked salmon, sliced or cut into chunks
3 tablespoons chopped dill, divided

1. Pour 1 cup of water into the inner pot. Arrange the potato slices as evenly as possible in a steaming basket and place the basket in the pot.

2. Lock the lid into place. Select Pressure Cook or Manual, and adjust the pressure to High and the time to 4 minutes. After cooking, quick release the pressure. Unlock the lid. Remove the basket, sprinkle the potatoes with ¼ teaspoon of salt, and set aside to cool. Empty the pot.

3. In a large bowl, make the custard by whisking the eggs, milk, cream, pepper, and the remaining ½ teaspoon of salt.

4. Grease the bottom and sides of a 1-quart, high-sided round dish with a teaspoon or so of the melted butter. Lay a third of the potatoes on the base and spread half the salmon and 1 tablespoon of dill over the potatoes. Top with another third of the potatoes, then the remaining salmon and 1 tablespoon of dill. Layer the rest of the potatoes on top.

5. Pour the custard over the potatoes, salmon, and dill; it should just come up to the top layer of the potatoes but not cover them. (You may not need all the custard.)

6. Preheat the broiler.

7. Add 1 cup of water to the inner pot and place a trivet inside. Cover the dish with aluminum foil and place it on the trivet. Lock the lid into place. Select Pressure Cook or Manual, and adjust the pressure to high and the time to 15 minutes. After cooking, let the pressure release naturally for 10 minutes, then quick release any remaining pressure.

8. Unlock the lid. Drizzle the remaining butter over the top of the potatoes and place the dish under the broiler for 3 to 5 minutes, or until the potatoes are lightly browned. Let sit for at least 10 minutes before serving warm, garnished with the remaining 1 tablespoon of dill and more pepper.

Mini Modification: You may need to use a smaller dish to fit in the Mini. If so, simply cut back on the amount of ingredients in the layers if necessary. The cook time will remain the same.

Use It Up: Leftover smoked salmon can be added to risotto or quiche. Use leftover dill in the Cod and Green Beans with Dill Mustard Sauce (page 94) or the Beet Salad with Creamy Dill Dressing (page 44).

Farfalle with Salmon, Fennel, and Tomatoes

I love the combination of fennel and tomatoes with salmon. In this recipe, I use the trio in a pasta dish with a light but creamy sauce. The fennel is subtle; if you like a more pronounced flavor, add a pinch of fennel seed, or chop the fronds and use as a garnish.

8 to 10 ounces center-cut salmon fillet

1 teaspoon kosher salt, divided

5 ounces farfalle pasta

½ pint cherry tomatoes, halved, divided

½ fennel head, trimmed and thinly sliced

2 garlic cloves, minced (about 2 teaspoons)

2 tablespoons extra-virgin olive oil

1¼ cups water

Nonstick cooking spray

¼ heavy (whipping) cream

½ teaspoon freshly ground black pepper

SERVES 2

PREP & FINISHING:
12 MINUTES

PRESSURE COOK:
5 MINUTES LOW

RELEASE:
QUICK

TOTAL TIME:
25 MINUTES

Per Serving
Calories: 713; Fat: 36 g;
Carbohydrates: 60 g;
Fiber: 6 g; Protein: 34 g;
Sodium: 407 mg

1. Sprinkle the salmon on both sides with ¼ teaspoon of salt and set aside.

2. Place the pasta in the inner pot. Add half the tomatoes, the fennel, garlic, olive oil, the remaining ¾ teaspoon of salt, and water, and stir gently.

3. Tear off a piece of aluminum foil large enough to completely enclose the salmon. Spray the foil with the cooking spray and wrap the salmon loosely in it. Place the salmon on top of the pasta. (If you have a trivet tall enough to clear the pasta, you can place the salmon on that.)

4. Lock the lid into place. Select Pressure Cook or Manual, and adjust the pressure to Low and the time to 5 minutes. After cooking, quick release the pressure.

5. Unlock the lid. Remove the salmon and place on a cutting board.

6. Stir the cream and the remaining tomatoes into the pasta. Test a piece of pasta; if it's not quite done, select Sauté, adjust to Medium heat, and bring the mixture to a simmer for a couple of minutes. Stir in the pepper.

7. Meanwhile, unwrap the salmon and discard the foil. Use a fork to break the salmon into bite-size chunks. If it is not quite done in the middle, add the fish to the simmering sauce for a minute or two until it's done. If it is done, add right before serving.

Lux Modification: In step 4, reduce the cooking time to 4 minutes.

Make It Dairy-Free: Omit the heavy cream; instead, stir in an extra tablespoon of extra-virgin olive oil and 1 to 2 tablespoons of water.

Use It Up: Use the other half of the fennel bulb in the Chicken Thighs with Salami and Fennel (page 110).

Cod and Green Beans with Dill Mustard Sauce

I'm generally not a big fan of cooking frozen meat in the Instant Pot®, but frozen fish fillets are a different story. Fish cooks so quickly that a pressure cooker can overcook it if you're not careful. In this recipe, the fish and beans cook at the same time, and you can give them an elegant finish with a quick and delicious sauce.

SERVES 2

PREP & FINISHING:
10 MINUTES

PRESSURE COOK:
3 MINUTES LOW

SAUTÉ:
3 MINUTES

RELEASE:
QUICK

TOTAL TIME:
25 MINUTES

Per Serving
Calories: 196; Fat: 7 g;
Carbohydrates: 10 g;
Fiber: 4 g; Protein: 23 g;
Sodium: 320 mg

2 (5- to 6-ounce) frozen cod fillets

½ teaspoon plus ⅛ teaspoon kosher salt, divided

6 ounces green beans, trimmed and cut into 2-inch pieces

2 tablespoons white wine

1 teaspoon crushed or minced garlic

1 tablespoon Dijon-style mustard

2 tablespoons heavy (whipping) cream

2 tablespoons chopped fresh dill, divided

1. Sprinkle the frozen fish fillets with ½ teaspoon of salt, and let them sit at room temperature while you prep the remaining ingredients.

2. Add 1 cup of water to the inner pot and stir in the remaining ⅛ teaspoon of salt. Add the beans to the water. Place the trivet inside the pot. Place the cod fillets on the trivet or in a steaming basket on the trivet.

3. Lock the lid into place. Select Pressure Cook or Manual, and adjust the pressure to Low and the time to 3 minutes. After cooking, quick release the pressure. Unlock the lid. Drain the beans into a colander. Cover the fish and beans with aluminum foil to keep warm.

4. Pour out any remaining water in the pot and return it to the base. Select Sauté and adjust to High heat. Pour the white wine into the pot and add the garlic. Bring to a simmer, then stir in the mustard and cream. Bring to a simmer and let cook for 1 minute. Stir in 1 tablespoon of dill.

5. Place the cod and beans on plates and spoon the sauce over. Garnish with the remaining 1 tablespoon of dill.

Lux Modification: In step 3, reduce the cooking time to 2 minutes. Check the fish with a fork; if it's not quite done, place the lid on the pot without locking it and wait for another minute.

Use It Up: Use leftover dill in the Scalloped Potatoes with Smoked Salmon (page 90). Leftover beans can be used in the Warm Thai-Style Green Bean and Tomato Salad (page 50).

Clam Chowder

Clam chowder is a go-to meal for the pressure cooker. While steaming your own clams isn't difficult, it is time consuming, so for a weeknight dinner, I use canned clams. A few slices of bread and a salad make it a great light dinner.

2 bacon slices, diced

½ small onion, chopped

1 celery rib, chopped

1 teaspoon all-purpose flour

¼ cup white wine, such as Sauvignon Blanc

4 ounces (½ cup) clam juice

½ cup water

2 (6-ounce) cans chopped clams, drained and liquid reserved

8 ounces red or gold potatoes, peeled and cut into 1-inch chunks

1 teaspoon dried thyme

1 bay leaf

¾ cup half-and-half

SERVES 2

PREP & FINISHING:
10 MINUTES

SAUTÉ:
7 MINUTES

PRESSURE COOK:
4 MINUTES HIGH

RELEASE:
NATURAL
5 MINUTES,
THEN QUICK

TOTAL TIME:
35 MINUTES

Per Serving
Calories: 438; Fat: 17 g;
Carbohydrates: 30 g;
Fiber: 4 g; Protein: 35 g;
Sodium: 1994 mg

1. Select Sauté and adjust to Medium heat. Place the bacon in the inner pot and cook, stirring, until the bacon is crisp and the fat is rendered, about 5 minutes. Transfer the bacon to a paper towel-lined plate to drain. Set aside.

2. Add the onion and celery to the pot and cook, stirring, until the vegetables begin to soften, about 1 minute. Add the flour and stir to coat the vegetables. Pour in the wine and bring to a simmer, cooking for about 1 minute or until the liquid is reduced by about a third. Add the clam juice, water, the liquid from the clams (but not the clams), potatoes, thyme, and bay leaf.

3. Lock the lid into place. Select Pressure Cook or Manual, and adjust the pressure to High and the time to 4 minutes. After cooking, let the pressure release naturally for 5 minutes, then quick release any remaining pressure.

4. Unlock the lid. Remove and discard the bay leaf. Stir in the clams and half-and-half. Select Sauté and adjust to Medium heat. Bring the soup to a simmer to heat the clams through. Ladle into bowls and sprinkle the bacon on top.

Double It: You can double this without any changes in cooking time. The bonus is that you can use up the whole bottle of clam juice (they are usually 8 ounces).

Make It Dairy-Free: Dairy-free clam chowder is usually tomato-based, as in Manhattan clam chowder. Omit the half-and-half, and add half a 14-ounce can of diced tomatoes with their juices with the clam juice and potatoes.

Make It Gluten-Free: Omit the flour; the soup will be slightly thinner, but still delicious.

Shrimp and Grits

When I moved to the South, I discovered that there's almost endless variation in shrimp and grits. My version is based on one in Savannah Seasons *by Elizabeth Terry. The sauce pressure cooks at the same time as the grits and then the shrimp are stirred in so they don't overcook.*

SERVES 2

PREP & FINISHING:
12 MINUTES

SAUTÉ:
8 MINUTES

PRESSURE COOK:
15 MINUTES HIGH

RELEASE:
NATURAL
10 MINUTES,
THEN QUICK

TOTAL TIME:
55 MINUTES

Per Serving
Calories: 512; Fat: 21 g;
Carbohydrates: 39 g;
Fiber: 2 g; Protein: 40 g;
Sodium: 1245 mg

3 bacon slices, diced

4 ounces white button or cremini mushrooms, washed and quartered

¼ cup diced onion

½ cup dry sherry

½ cup brewed coffee

¾ cup tomato juice

1 tablespoon all-purpose flour

1 teaspoon dried thyme

1 to 2 teaspoons hot pepper sauce, such as Tabasco or Crystal

⅓ cup polenta or grits (not instant or quick-cook)

⅔ cup whole milk

⅔ cup low-sodium vegetable stock

¼ teaspoon kosher salt

1 tablespoon unsalted butter

8 ounces peeled and deveined raw medium or large shrimp (halved if large)

1. Select Sauté and adjust to Medium heat. Add the bacon to the inner pot and cook, stirring, until it is crisp and the fat has rendered, about 4 minutes. Using a slotted spoon, remove the bacon and place on a paper towel–lined plate. Set aside.

2. Add the mushrooms and onion and stir to coat with the fat. Add the sherry and coffee and scrape up any browned bits on the bottom of the pot. Let simmer for about 4 minutes, or until the liquid is reduced by about half.

3. In a small bowl, add the tomato juice. Stir the flour into the tomato juice, and then pour the mixture into the inner pot. Add the thyme and hot sauce, and stir to combine. Place a trivet in the pot that's tall enough to clear the mushroom mixture.

4. In a heat-proof bowl that holds at least 4 cups, add the polenta, milk, stock, and salt. Stir. Place the bowl on top of the trivet.

5. Lock the lid into place. Select Pressure Cook or Manual, and adjust the pressure to High and the time to 15 minutes. After cooking, let the pressure release naturally for 10 minutes, then quick release any remaining pressure.

6. Unlock the lid. Carefully remove the bowl of polenta. Add the butter to the bowl and stir to melt the butter and any lumps in the polenta. Taste and adjust seasoning. Set aside.

7. Add the shrimp to the pot. Select Sauté and adjust to Medium heat. Simmer for about 4 minutes, or until the shrimp are cooked through. Stir in the bacon.

8. To serve, divide the grits between two bowls and top with the shrimp mixture.

Make It Gluten-Free: Omit the flour in the sauce. After pressure cooking, whisk together 1 tablespoon of cornstarch with 2 tablespoons of water. Stir into the sauce while the shrimp cook.

Cilantro-Coconut Shrimp and Broccoli

I got the idea for this dish from a Food & Wine *magazine recipe, though the original recipe felt confusing and unnecessarily complicated. I kept the flavors, but streamlined the cooking process, and added noodles to make it a complete meal. It's important to use the right size shrimp and keep them cold right until they are cooked so they don't overcook.*

SERVES 2

PREP & FINISHING:
12 MINUTES

SAUTÉ:
2 MINUTES

PRESSURE COOK:
0 MINUTES LOW

RELEASE:
QUICK

TOTAL TIME:
20 MINUTES

Per Serving
Calories: 864; Fat: 51 g;
Carbohydrates: 59 g;
Fiber: 8 g; Protein: 46 g;
Sodium: 852 mg

1 (14-ounce) can coconut milk
2 cups loosely packed cilantro
1 jalapeño, seeded and cut
into chunks
1 scallion, green part only, cut
into chunks
1 garlic clove
1½ teaspoons kosher salt

¾ cup water
4 ounces Chinese wheat
noodles (I use KA-ME brand)
or 1 (4-ounce) package
ramen noodles
10 ounces peeled (about
21 to 25) shrimp, refrigerated
6 to 8 ounces broccoli florets

1. In a blender jar, add the coconut milk, cilantro, jalapeño, scallion, garlic, and salt. Blend until smooth. (Or place these ingredients in a deep, narrow container and use an immersion blender to purée.)

2. Pour the sauce into the inner pot and add the water. Select Sauté and adjust to High heat. Bring just to a simmer, then turn the Instant Pot® off.

3. Break up the noodles into 3 or 4 pieces and place them in the pot in a single layer as much as possible. Layer the shrimp and broccoli over the noodles.

4. Lock the lid into place. Select Pressure Cook or Manual, and adjust the pressure to Low and the time to 0 minutes. After cooking, quick release the pressure.

5. Unlock the lid. Gently stir the mixture until the broccoli and shrimp are coated with sauce. Ladle into bowls and serve immediately.

Make It Gluten-Free: Leave the noodles out and reduce the water to ¼ cup. Serve over Basic White or Brown Rice (page 163).

Lux Modification: In Step 2, bring the sauce to a full boil and then follow the rest of the directions as written.

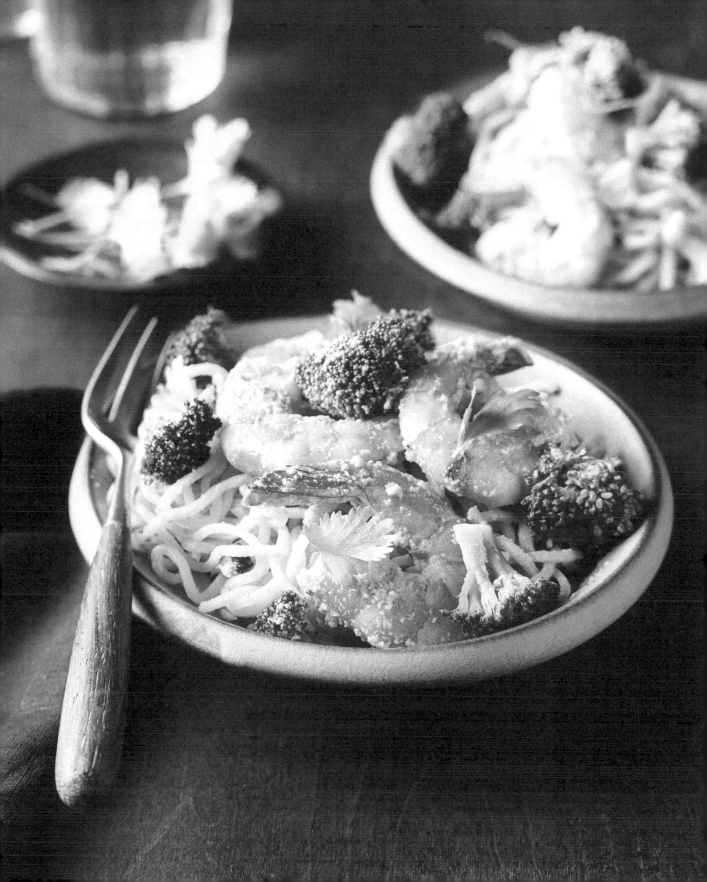

Italian Tuna and Bean Salad

White beans and tuna are a classic Italian combination, served warm with pasta or at room temperature in a salad. I like to add green beans and toma-toes to make a light and satisfying lunch or dinner. If you don't have capers on hand, you can substitute pitted Kalamata or similar olives.

SERVES 2

PREP & FINISHING:
10 MINUTES

PRESSURE COOK:
7 MINUTES HIGH
THEN 0 MINUTES
HIGH

RELEASE:
NATURAL
5 MINUTES,
THEN QUICK
THEN QUICK

TOTAL TIME:
35 MINUTES

Per Serving
Calories: 448; Fat: 27 g;
Carbohydrates: 29 g;
Fiber: 10 g; Protein: 28 g;
Sodium: 537 mg

2 ounces dry cannellini beans (about ⅓ cup)

3 cups water, divided

2 teaspoons kosher salt, divided

6 ounces green beans, washed, trimmed, and cut into 1-inch pieces

1 (6-ounce) can oil-packed tuna, drained

½ cup cherry or grape tomatoes halves

1 tablespoon capers, drained

2 tablespoons chopped red onion

2 tablespoons chiffonade-cut fresh basil

For the dressing

2 tablespoons extra-virgin olive oil

1 tablespoon red wine vinegar

½ teaspoon kosher salt

¼ teaspoon granulated garlic or garlic powder

¼ teaspoon coarsely ground black pepper

1. Pour the beans into a small bowl. Add 2 cups of water and 1½ tea-spoons of salt. Let soak for 6 to 8 hours. Drain and rinse.

2. Add the soaked beans to the inner pot. Add 1 cup of water and the remaining ½ teaspoon of salt. Lock the lid into place. Select Pressure Cook or Manual, and adjust the pressure to High and the time to 7 minutes.

3. While the beans are cooking, chop the vegetables for the salad and prepare the dressing. To make the dressing, whisk all of the ingredients in a small bowl, or place them in a small jar with a tight-fitting lid, and shake to combine.

4. After cooking, let the pressure release naturally for 5 minutes, then quick release any remaining pressure.

5. Unlock the lid. Drain the beans in a strainer or colander, then transfer to a medium bowl. Shake or whisk the dressing and pour it over the beans. Wipe out the inner pot and return it to the base.

6. Place the green beans in a steamer basket. Add 1 cup of water to the inner pot and place the steamer basket inside. Lock the lid into place. Select Steam and adjust pressure to High and time to 0 minutes. After cooking, quick release the pressure.

7. Unlock the lid. Add the green beans to the cannellini beans in the bowl and toss. Add the tuna, tomatoes, capers, onion, and basil to the bowl. Toss gently and serve.

Double It: Double the cannellini beans and use the extra in Minestrone (page 74) or any recipe calling for canned beans. Double the green beans and refrigerate half to use in the Warm Thai-Style Green Bean and Tomato Salad (page 50).

Use It Up: Use the remaining cherry tomatoes in the Warm Thai-Style Green Bean and Tomato Salad (page 50), the Greek Salad with Bulgur Wheat (page 62), or the Farfalle with Salmon, Fennel, and Tomatoes (page 92). Use the remaining basil in the Thai Red Curry Beef (page 129) or the Warm Thai-Style Green Bean and Tomato Salad (page 50).

Perfect Chicken Breast

If you read through many of my chicken recipes in this cookbook, you'll notice that most call for thighs. That's because they're so versatile; depending on how they're cut, they can adapt to a wide variety of cooking times. Boneless, skinless chicken breasts are trickier, but if you're cooking for a white meat fan, all is not lost! Cook them separately and cut them up, then add to them to Chicken Paprikash (page 112), Creamy Salsa Verde Chicken (page 105), or Sweet and Sour Chicken (page 114). Each of those recipes include tips to let you know how to adjust your recipe for the addition of chicken breast.

SERVES 4

PREP & FINISHING:
2 MINUTES

MANUAL:
5 MINUTES LOW

RELEASE:
NATURAL
8 MINUTES,
THEN QUICK

TOTAL TIME:
20 MINUTES

Per Serving
Calories: 240; Fat: 3 g;
Carbohydrates: 0 g;
Fiber: 0 g; Protein: 52 g;
Sodium: 299 mg

1 (16-ounce) boneless, skinless chicken breast

½ teaspoon kosher salt

1 cup water

1. Salt the chicken breast on both sides.

2. Pour 1 cup of water into the inner pot. Place the chicken breast on a trivet or shallow steamer basket and place in the pot.

3. Lock the lid in place. Select Pressure Cook or Manual, and adjust the pressure to Low and the time to 5 minutes. After cooking, let the pressure release naturally for 8 minutes, then quick release any remaining pressure.

4. Unlock the lid. Remove the chicken to a plate or rack. Use a thermometer to test the temperature; the breasts should register at least 150°F in the center (residual heat will bring the temperature up). If not, return the chicken to the pot, place the lid back on, and let the chicken steam for an additional 3 to 4 minutes.

Lux Modification: In step 3, keep the cooking time the same, but quick release the pressure after 5 minutes.

Use It Up: Not only can you use the cooked chicken breast in some of the recipes in this chapter, but it's great cut up for lunchtime salads or sandwiches.

Creamy Salsa Verde Chicken

This is a dead simple and deliciously creamy salsa verde chicken recipe. You can also use about half the sauce mixed with the chicken for a taco or quesadilla filling. Jump to the tip for yet another variation: a Mexican-inspired soup.

10 ounces (2 to 3) boneless, skinless chicken thighs

1½ cups tomatillo-based green salsa (I like Frontera brand)

½ cup heavy (whipping) cream

½ cup shredded Monterey Jack cheese

1 cup cooked Basic White Rice (page 163)

1. Place the chicken in the inner pot and add the salsa.

2. Lock the lid in place. Select Pressure Cook or Manual, and adjust the pressure to High and the time to 8 minutes. After cooking, let the pressure release naturally for 5 minutes, then quick release any remaining pressure.

3. Unlock the lid. Remove the chicken to a sheet pan or bowl and let cool for a few minutes. Stir the cream into the sauce in the pot. Keep the sauce warm. When ready to serve, stir in the cheese.

4. When the chicken is just cool enough to handle, cut or pull it into small chunks. Finish the dish by mixing the chicken back into the cheesy sauce. Serve it over the rice.

For Chicken Breast Lovers: Follow the directions on page 104 for Perfect Chicken Breast. Use just 1 (4- to 5-ounce) chicken thigh, then after cooking, add 5 to 6 ounces of cooked chicken breast.

Use It Up: Extra Monterey Jack cheese can be used in the Chorizo and Green Chile Breakfast Casserole (page 32).

Variation: For a Mexican-inspired soup, when the chicken is added back to the pot in step 4, add ½ cup or so of chicken stock, ½ cup of frozen corn, ½ cup of canned (drained) or Basic Beans (page 162), and ½ cup of cooked Basic White or Brown Rice (page 163). Select Sauté and adjust to Medium heat. Let the soup come to a simmer, then top with diced tomatoes, more cheese, and tortilla chips.

SERVES 2

PREP & FINISHING:
5 MINUTES

PRESSURE COOK:
8 MINUTES HIGH

RELEASE:
NATURAL
5 MINUTES,
THEN QUICK

TOTAL TIME:
25 MINUTES,
PLUS VARIOUS
FINISHING
TIMES

Per Serving
Calories: 605; Fat: 36 g;
Carbohydrates: 31 g;
Fiber: 1 g; Protein: 37 g;
Sodium: 469 mg

Shawarma-Style Chicken and Rice

Traditional shawarma is seasoned meat—originally lamb, but beef or chicken made a later appearance—grilled on a spit, then served on pita bread. In the States, the term gets used for any meat cooked with vaguely Middle Eastern spices. I don't claim that this dish is shawarma, but it's inspired by the traditional flavors of the grilled meats, and is just as delicious.

SERVES 2

PREP & FINISHING:
10 MINUTES

PRESSURE COOK:
4 MINUTES HIGH

RELEASE:
NATURAL
10 MINUTES,
THEN QUICK

TOTAL TIME:
35 MINUTES, PLUS
MARINATING TIME

Per Serving
Calories: 505; Fat: 22 g;
Carbohydrates: 41 g;
Fiber: 2 g; Protein: 37 g;
Sodium: 379 mg

12 ounces boneless, skinless chicken thighs
¾ teaspoon kosher salt, divided
2 tablespoons extra-virgin olive oil
2 tablespoons plain Greek yogurt
2 tablespoons freshly squeezed lemon juice
3 garlic cloves, minced (about 3 teaspoons)
1 teaspoon cumin

1 teaspoon smoked paprika
¼ teaspoon turmeric
¼ teaspoon allspice
¼ teaspoon cinnamon
¼ teaspoon freshly ground black pepper
¼ teaspoon red pepper flakes
½ cup long-grain white rice, rinsed
½ cup water
1 tablespoon chopped fresh parsley (optional)

1. Sprinkle the chicken thighs on both sides with ½ teaspoon of salt. Place in a resealable plastic bag and set aside while you mix the marinade.

2. In a small bowl, mix the olive oil, yogurt, lemon juice, garlic, cumin, paprika, turmeric, allspice, cinnamon, pepper, and red pepper flakes, until thoroughly combined. Pour the marinade into the bag over the chicken and manipulate the chicken to coat it with the sauce. Set aside for as long as you can—20 minutes is fine; an hour is better.

3. Place the rice in the inner pot. Add the water and the remaining ¼ teaspoon of salt, and stir to dissolve the salt. Remove the chicken thighs from the marinade and place on top of the rice. Drizzle the marinade over the chicken.

4. Lock the lid into place. Select Pressure Cook or Manual, and adjust the pressure to High and the time to 4 minutes. When cooking is complete, let the pressure release naturally for 10 minutes, then quick release any remaining pressure.

5. Unlock the lid. Serve sprinkled with parsley (if using).

Make Ahead: You can marinate the chicken in the morning before you leave for work.

Make It Dairy-Free: You can leave the yogurt out of the marinade; the sauce won't be as thick but will still be delicious.

Spicy Chicken Lettuce Cups

Ever since the restaurant P.F. Chang's put them on the menu, recipes for "copycat" chicken lettuce wraps have exploded all over the Internet. I've never actually tried the restaurant version, so I can't say if this is similar, but I can say that it's fast and delicious. If you chop the vegetables while the chicken cooks, it's even faster.

SERVES 2

PREP & FINISHING:
10 MINUTES

PRESSURE COOK:
7 MINUTES HIGH

RELEASE:
QUICK

SAUTÉ:
8 MINUTES

TOTAL TIME:
35 MINUTES

Per Serving
Calories: 387; Fat: 15 g;
Carbohydrates: 26 g;
Fiber: 3 g; Protein: 36 g;
Sodium: 1150 mg

12 ounces boneless, skinless chicken thighs
2 tablespoons Chicken Stock (page 158)
2 tablespoons rice vinegar
3 tablespoons hoisin sauce
1 tablespoon soy sauce
2 teaspoons chili-garlic sauce or Sriracha
2 teaspoons minced garlic
2 teaspoons minced fresh ginger
2 tablespoons minced jalapeño

½ cup chopped water chestnuts
½ cup chopped red bell pepper
2 scallions, chopped, green and white parts separated
1 small butter or Boston lettuce head
1 tablespoon toasted sesame oil
¼ cup toasted chopped almonds or peanuts, for garnish (optional)
2 tablespoons coarsely chopped cilantro, for garnish (optional)

1. Place the chicken thighs in the inner pot. Add the chicken stock, vinegar, hoisin, soy sauce, chili-garlic sauce, garlic, and ginger. Stir gently to combine. Lock the lid into place. Select Pressure Cook or Manual, and adjust the pressure to High and the time to 7 minutes. When cooking is complete, quick release the pressure.

2. Unlock and the lid. Remove the chicken thighs to a cutting board.

3. Add the jalapeño, water chestnuts, red pepper, and the white scallion part to the sauce in the pot. Select Sauté and adjust to Medium heat. Bring to a simmer and cook, stirring occasionally, until the vegetables have softened somewhat and the sauce has thickened, 6 to 8 minutes.

4. While the vegetables cook, chop the chicken into small pieces, discarding any fat or gristle. Separate the lettuce leaves, discarding any tough outer leaves and setting aside the small inner leaves for another use. You'll want 6 to 10 leaves, depending on size and your appetites.

5. Add the chicken and the sesame oil to the vegetables in the pot and stir to rewarm the chicken.

6. To serve, spoon some of the chicken into each of the lettuce leaves. Top with the scallion greens and the nuts and cilantro (if using).

Double It: This doubles easily; leftovers will keep for several days in the refrigerator. Double all the ingredients except the chicken stock.

Easier Together: While the chicken cooks, both partners can chop the vegetables. Afterward, one partner can cook the sauce and vegetables while the other chops the chicken and prepares the lettuce.

Use It Up: Use the extra water chestnuts in the Rice Pilaf with Bacon and Chestnuts (page 64). Use the rest of the bell pepper in the Thai Red Curry Beef (page 129), Southwestern Black Bean Salad (page 60), or the salsa for the Pork Tacos with Pineapple Salsa (page 138).

Chicken Thighs with Salami and Fennel

This dish is based on a recipe I first saw in The New York Times, *which was inspired by a recipe from New Orleans chef Donald Link. If it sounds weird to cook chicken with salami, I assure you that it's delicious. Ask at the deli counter for a salami that's not too hard; cotto salami is a good choice.*

SERVES 2

PREP & FINISHING:
15 MINUTES

SAUTÉ:
10 MINUTES

PRESSURE COOK:
10 MINUTES HIGH

RELEASE:
NATURAL
5 MINUTES,
THEN QUICK

TOTAL TIME:
50 MINUTES

Per Serving
Calories: 486; Fat: 34 g;
Carbohydrates: 11 g;
Fiber: 4 g; Protein: 24 g;
Sodium: 1235 mg

2 large or 4 small bone-in, skin-on chicken thighs

½ teaspoon kosher salt

2 tablespoons extra-virgin olive oil

½ fennel bulb, trimmed and cut into ¼-inch wedges

½ small onion, sliced

½ cup dry red or white wine

½ (14-ounce) can diced tomatoes

¼ cup diced salami

½ cup Chicken Stock (page 158)

1 tablespoon red wine vinegar

1 tablespoon Dijon-style mustard

1. Sprinkle the chicken thighs on both sides with the salt.

2. Select Sauté and adjust to High heat. Add the olive oil to the pot and heat until it shimmers, Add the chicken thighs, skin-side down, and let them cook, undisturbed, for about 5 minutes, or until the skin is golden brown and most of the fat under the skin has rendered out. Turn the thighs to the other side and cook for about 2 minutes. Remove the thighs and set aside.

3. Carefully pour off almost all the fat in the pot, leaving about 2 tablespoons in it. Add the fennel and onion, and stir to coat with the fat. Cook without stirring until the vegetables begin to brown, about 2 minutes.

4. Add the wine and scrape the bottom of the pot to release the browned bits. Simmer for about 4 minutes, or until the liquid reduces by half. Add the tomatoes, salami, stock, vinegar, and mustard. Stir to combine. Add the chicken thighs, skin-side up, to the pot.

5. Lock the lid in place. Select Pressure Cook or Manual, and adjust the pressure to High and the time to 10 minutes. After cooking, release the pressure naturally for 5 minutes, then quick release any remaining pressure. While the pressure releases, preheat the oven to broil.

6. Unlock the lid. Remove the chicken thighs and blot them dry. Place them on a rack placed over a sheet pan or baking sheet. Place the pan in the oven on the top or second rack (depending on the strength of your broiler). Broil for 3 to 5 minutes, or until browned.

7. Continue with the sauce while the chicken crisps. Spoon or blot the fat from the top of the sauce. If you like a thicker sauce, simmer it on Sauté for a few minutes while the chicken crisps. To serve, ladle a spoonful of sauce on each plate and top with a spoonful of vegetables and a chicken thigh (this keeps the skin crisper than putting the sauce over the chicken).

Easier Together: You'll save time if one cook salts and browns the chicken while the other person slices the vegetables.

Mini Modification: You'll probably have to brown the chicken in two batches, which will increase the prep time.

Use It Up: The other half of the fennel bulb can be used in the Farfalle with Salmon, Fennel, and Tomatoes (page 92). The remaining canned tomatoes can be used with Easy Chili (page 123) or Chicken Paprikash (page 112).

Chicken Paprikash

There are probably as many recipes for chicken paprikash as there are cooks in Hungary. I've tried a few versions and they're all delicious, but I wanted something faster. The flavors of my recipe are fairly traditional, but pressure cooking everything—noodles and all—is my own twist.

12 ounces boneless, skinless
    chicken thighs
¼ teaspoon kosher salt
4 ounces wide egg noodles
1 small onion, sliced
½ (14-ounce) can diced
    tomatoes, with its juices

1 Hungarian wax pepper,
    Anaheim pepper, or small red
    bell pepper, seeded and cut
    into chunks
2 tablespoons paprika
1½ cups low-sodium
    chicken stock
⅓ cup sour cream

SERVES 2

PREP & FINISHING:
10 MINUTES

PRESSURE COOK:
5 MINUTES HIGH

RELEASE:
QUICK

TOTAL TIME:
25 MINUTES

Per Serving
Calories: 564; Fat: 18 g;
Carbohydrates: 56 g;
Fiber: 7 g; Protein: 45 g;
Sodium: 488 mg

1. Cut the chicken thighs into bite-sized pieces and sprinkle with the salt. Let the pieces sit while you chop the vegetables.

2. Place the noodles in the bottom of the inner pot. Add the chicken, onion, tomatoes, and pepper.

3. Stir the paprika into the chicken stock and pour it over the ingredients in the pot. Ensure the noodles are covered with the liquid.

4. Lock the lid into place. Select Pressure Cook or Manual, adjust the pressure to High and the time to 5 minutes. After cooking, quick release the pressure.

5. Unlock the lid. Let the chicken and noodles rest for a minute or so, until the sauce is barely simmering. Stir in the sour cream.

For Chicken Breast Lovers: Follow the directions on page 104 for Perfect Chicken Breast. Use just 1 (4- to 5-ounce) chicken thigh, then after cooking, add 5 to 6 ounces of chopped cooked chicken breast.

Use It Up: Use the other half of the tomatoes in Easy Chili (page 123).

Teriyaki Chicken and Rice

If you've never made your own teriyaki sauce, this recipe may be an eye-opener. Sweet and savory with complex flavors, this chicken and rice dish is a breeze to make. It's even easier if you can find frozen minced garlic and ginger cubes, which work perfectly in this sauce.

12 ounces boneless, skinless chicken thighs

¼ cup soy sauce

3 tablespoons honey

1 tablespoon rice vinegar

1 tablespoon rice wine or dry sherry

2 teaspoons minced fresh ginger

2 garlic cloves, minced or pressed (about 2 teaspoons)

½ cup long-grain white rice, rinsed

½ cup water

¼ teaspoon kosher salt

1 tablespoon toasted sesame seeds, for garnish (optional)

SERVES 2

PREP & FINISHING:
10 MINUTES

PRESSURE COOK:
4 MINUTES HIGH

RELEASE:
NATURAL
10 MINUTES,
THEN QUICK

TOTAL TIME:
35 MINUTES

Per Serving
Calories: 496; Fat: 7 g;
Carbohydrates: 70 g;
Fiber: 1 g; Protein: 38 g;
Sodium: 1198 mg

1. Place the chicken in a resealable plastic bag and set aside while you mix the teriyaki sauce.

2. In a small bowl, mix the soy sauce, honey, vinegar, rice wine, ginger, and garlic until thoroughly combined. Pour the marinade over the chicken in the bag and manipulate the chicken to coat it with the sauce. Set aside for as long as you can—20 minutes is fine; an hour is better.

3. Pour the rice into the inner pot. Add the water and salt, and stir to dissolve the salt. Remove the chicken thighs from the marinade and place them on top of the rice. Drizzle a tablespoon or so of the teriyaki sauce over the chicken.

4. Lock the lid into place. Select Pressure Cook or Manual, and adjust the pressure to High and the time to 4 minutes. When cooking is complete, let the pressure release naturally for 10 minutes, then quick release any remaining pressure.

5. Unlock the lid. Serve sprinkled with the sesame seeds (if using).

Make It Gluten-Free: Use gluten-free tamari in place of the soy sauce.

Sweet and Sour Chicken

In Chinese-American restaurants, most sweet and sour chicken starts with battered and deep-fried chicken, and often ends with a too sweet, too thick sauce. While I have nothing against deep-fried chicken, sometimes it's nice to have a lighter dish, and that's when this recipe is a perfect choice.

SERVES 2

PREP & FINISHING:
10 MINUTES

PRESSURE COOK:
5 MINUTES HIGH

RELEASE:
QUICK

SAUTÉ:
5 MINUTES

TOTAL TIME:
30 MINUTES

Per Serving
Calories: 321; Fat: 7 g;
Carbohydrates: 29 g;
Fiber: 2 g; Protein: 35 g;
Sodium: 773 mg

12 ounces boneless skinless chicken thighs, cut into 1-inch chunks
2 tablespoons rice vinegar
2 tablespoons ketchup
2 tablespoons low-sodium chicken stock
2 tablespoons brown sugar
1 tablespoon soy sauce
1 teaspoon freshly grated ginger
1 red bell pepper, seeded, cut into 1-inch chunks
1 cup (¾-inch) pineapple chunks

1. Place the chicken thighs in the inner pot. Add the vinegar, ketchup, chicken stock, brown sugar, soy sauce, and ginger. Stir gently to combine and dissolve the sugar.

2. Lock the lid into place. Select Pressure Cook or Manual, and adjust the pressure to High and the time to 5 minutes. When cooking is complete, quick release the pressure.

3. Unlock the lid. Add the bell pepper and pineapple to the sauce in the pot. Select Sauté and adjust to Medium heat. Bring to a simmer and cook, stirring occasionally, until the peppers have softened somewhat and the sauce has thickened, 5 to 6 minutes.

4. Serve over rice, if desired.

For Chicken Breast Lovers: Follow the directions on page 104 for Perfect Chicken Breast. Use just 1 (4- to 5-ounce) chicken thigh, then after cooking, add 5 to 6 ounces of cooked, chopped chicken breast.

Use It Up: Use the any leftover pineapple in the Pork Tacos with Pineapple Salsa (page 138).

Chicken Noodle Soup

I firmly believe that the only way to make good chicken soup is to make a really good chicken stock first. For most recipes, I'm all for using commercial chicken stock or broth, but not for chicken soup. And all those recipes that say you can make the broth by cooking a chicken and then use the meat for the soup? They're wrong. By the time you have flavorful broth, you have tasteless, overcooked chicken. So, if you want chicken noodle soup, plan ahead and make Chicken Stock (page 158) first. You'll never look back.

1 tablespoon extra-virgin olive oil or vegetable oil

1 small onion, chopped

1 teaspoon minced garlic (1 small clove)

1 large parsley sprig, stemmed, leaves separated and chopped

1 bay leaf

3 cups Chicken Stock (page 158)

½ teaspoon kosher salt

1 (12-ounce) boneless, skinless chicken breast

1 large carrot, peeled and cut into ¼-inch rounds

1 celery rib, sliced ¼ inch thick

2 ounces egg noodles (about 1½ cups)

SERVES 2

PREP & FINISHING:
10 MINUTES

SAUTÉ:
3 MINUTES

PRESSURE COOK:
5 MINUTES HIGH

RELEASE:
QUICK

TOTAL TIME:
25 MINUTES

Per Serving
Calories: 373; Fat: 12 g;
Carbohydrates: 17 g;
Fiber: 3 g; Protein: 49 g;
Sodium: 460 mg

1. Select Sauté and adjust to Medium heat. Add the oil to the pot and heat until it shimmers. Add the onion and cook, stirring often, for about 2 minutes. Add the garlic, parsley stem, and bay leaf and cook for 30 seconds, or until fragrant. Add the chicken stock and salt. Add the chicken breast, carrot, celery, and egg noodles.

2. Lock the lid into place. Select Pressure Cook or Manual, and adjust the pressure to High and the time to 5 minutes. After cooking, quick release any remaining pressure.

3. Unlock the lid. Use tongs to remove the chicken breast and place it on a cutting board. Cut it into bite-size pieces. If the center of the chicken is not completely cooked, return those pieces to the soup and bring to a simmer for a couple of minutes until the chicken is cooked through.

4. Remove the bay leaf and parsley stem. Return the remaining chicken to the soup. Taste and adjust the seasoning. Garnish with the parsley leaves.

Use It Up: You can use extra egg noodles in Chicken Paprikash (page 112) and the parsley in Greek Salad with Bulgur Wheat (page 62).

Barbecue Chicken Sandwiches with Slaw

I know this looks like a long recipe, but if the two of you work together, it goes quickly. The sauce is so much better than bottled barbecue sauce and worth the time to make it. Even if you skip the slaw, the sandwiches are still great.

SERVES 2

PREP & FINISHING:
12 MINUTES

PRESSURE COOK:
8 MINUTES HIGH

RELEASE:
NATURAL
5 MINUTES,
THEN QUICK

TOTAL TIME:
35 MINUTES

Per Serving
Calories: 475; Fat: 14 g;
Carbohydrates: 49 g;
Fiber: 5 g; Protein: 40 g;
Sodium: 1323 mg

For the slaw

2 cups shredded cabbage or coleslaw mix

1 small carrot, peeled and shredded or grated

1 teaspoon kosher salt

1 teaspoon cider vinegar

2 tablespoons mayonnaise

⅛ teaspoon prepared horseradish

1 teaspoon brown sugar

⅛ teaspoon whole mustard seed

⅛ teaspoon whole celery seed

Pinch freshly ground black pepper

For the chicken

12 ounces boneless, skinless chicken thighs

½ teaspoon kosher salt

⅔ cup tomato sauce

½ small onion, cut into chunks

1 garlic clove

1 tablespoon ground ancho chile powder

1 tablespoon Dijon-style mustard

1 tablespoon cider or wine vinegar

2 tablespoons brown sugar

½ teaspoon Worcestershire sauce

1 chipotle chile in adobo sauce

2 hamburger buns, split

1. To start the slaw, place the cabbage and carrot in a salad spinner or colander and sprinkle with the salt. Toss gently and set aside to drain for 15 minutes while you start the chicken.

2. Sprinkle the chicken thighs with the salt and set aside.

3. Add the tomato sauce to the inner pot. Add the onion, garlic, chile powder, mustard, vinegar, brown sugar, Worcestershire sauce, and chipotle. Stir to combine. Place the chicken in the pot.

4. Lock the lid into place. Select Pressure Cook or Manual, and adjust the pressure to High and the time to 8 minutes.

5. While the chicken cooks, return to the slaw. In a medium bowl, whisk together the vinegar, mayonnaise, horseradish, brown sugar, mustard seed, whole celery seed, and pepper. When the cabbage and carrots have drained for 15 minutes, rinse and spin or pat dry. Add them to the dressing and toss to coat.

6. After cooking, let the pressure release naturally for 5 minutes, then quick release any remaining pressure.

7. Unlock the lid. Use tongs to remove the chicken thighs from the pot to a cutting board. Let cool for a few minutes, then chop or shred with two forks, discarding any fat or gristle.

8. Using an immersion blender, purée the sauce in the pot. Taste and adjust the seasoning. Return the chicken to the pot and stir to combine.

9. To serve, spoon the chicken onto the bottom halves of the buns. Finish with a scoop of slaw and the top bun (or serve the slaw on the side).

Easier Together: This is a perfect "divide and conquer" recipe—one person can make the slaw while the other one concentrates on the chicken.

Time Saver: Salting the cabbage and carrots makes for a nicer texture and keeps the slaw from weeping, but if you're pressed for time, you can skip it. Just add the salt to the dressing.

Use It Up: Use leftover cabbage in the Kielbasa and Vegetable Stew (page 131).

Turkey and Stuffing for Two

Who says you can't cook Thanksgiving turkey, gravy, and stuffing for two, without a ton of leftovers? This recipe does take some time, but it's a holiday, right? Besides, most of that is for making turkey stock, which can be done ahead of time. Depending on your market, you may find turkey tenderloins packed in a brine. That's fine, but you won't want to salt the tenderloin in that case.

SERVES 2

PREP & FINISHING:
10 MINUTES

SAUTÉ:
15 MINUTES

PRESSURE COOK:
90 MINUTES HIGH
THEN 5 MINUTES
HIGH *THEN*
7 MINUTES HIGH

RELEASE:
NATURAL
15 MINUTES,
THEN QUICK *THEN*
NATURAL
3 MINUTES,
THEN QUICK *THEN*
NATURAL
8 MINUTES,
THEN QUICK

TOTAL TIME:
2 HOURS
30 MINUTES

Per Serving
Calories: 536; Fat: 20 g;
Carbohydrates: 32 g;
Fiber: 2 g; Protein: 57 g;
Sodium: 505 mg

2 turkey wings or thighs (about 2 pounds)

1¼ teaspoons kosher salt, divided

3 cups water

1 (12-ounce) turkey tenderloin

2 teaspoons poultry seasoning

½ teaspoon crumbled dried sage

¼ teaspoon freshly ground black pepper

1 tablespoon unsalted butter

2 bacon slices, chopped

½ cup chopped onion

1 celery rib, diced

¼ cup dry sherry

3 cups stale white bread cubes, cut into 1-inch pieces (3 to 4 slices)

1 large egg

2 tablespoons all-purpose flour

1. Using the directions for the Chicken Stock on page 158, make stock using the turkey wings, ¼ teaspoon of salt, and the water. Let the stock cool. Spoon off the fat from the top of the stock. This should make about 3½ cups of stock. (This portion of the recipe takes about 2 hours, so plan accordingly.)

2. Sprinkle ½ teaspoon of salt over the turkey tenderloin. In a small bowl, mix the poultry seasoning, sage, and pepper. Rub 1 teaspoon of this mixture over the turkey and set the turkey aside.

3. Select Sauté and adjust to Medium heat. Add the butter to the inner pot. When it has melted, add the bacon and cook, stirring, until most of the fat has rendered, about 4 minutes. Add the onion and celery and cook, stirring, until the vegetables have softened, about 2 minutes. Pour in the sherry and stir to scrape up the browned bits off the bottom of the pot. Bring to a simmer and reduce the sherry by about half. Transfer the bacon and vegetable mixture to a medium bowl.

4. Add 2 cups of stock to the pot. With the heat still on Medium, bring the stock to a simmer and reduce it by half, so you have about 1 cup left.

5. While the stock reduces, add the bread cubes, ¼ teaspoon of salt, and 1 teaspoon of the reserved spice mixture to the bacon mixture. In a small bowl, whisk the egg into ½ cup of stock and pour that over the bread mixture. Stir gently until the bread has absorbed most of the liquid. Add another tablespoon or so of stock if the mixture is too dry. Transfer the stuffing to a 1-quart heat-proof bowl.

6. Leaving the reduced stock in the pot, place a trivet with handles in the pot and then place the bowl of stuffing on top.

7. Lock the lid into place. Select Pressure Cook or Manual, and adjust the pressure to High and the time to 5 minutes. After cooking, let the pressure release naturally for 3 minutes, then quick release any remaining pressure. Unlock the lid. Place the turkey tenderloin next to the stuffing on the trivet, or on top of the stuffing if there's not enough room next to it.

8. Lock the lid into place. Select Pressure Cook or Manual, and adjust the pressure to High and the time to 7 minutes. After cooking, let the pressure release naturally for 8 minutes, then quick release any remaining pressure.

9. Unlock the lid. Carefully remove the stuffing from the pot and cover it with aluminum foil. Transfer the turkey to a cutting board and tent it with foil.

10. Select Sauté and adjust to Medium heat. Bring the stock to a simmer.

11. In a small bowl, whisk together the flour with ¼ cup of the remaining stock. Stir in the remaining spice mixture and the remaining ¼ teaspoon of salt. Whisk the mixture into the stock in the pot and cook, stirring, for 2 to 3 minutes, or until the gravy is thickened.

12. As the gravy cooks, slice the turkey. Serve the turkey and stuffing with gravy.

Easier Together: One cook can season the turkey while the other person cooks the bacon and vegetables. Later, one can make the gravy while the other person slices the turkey.

Make Ahead: You can make the stock ahead of time and refrigerate for up to 3 days.

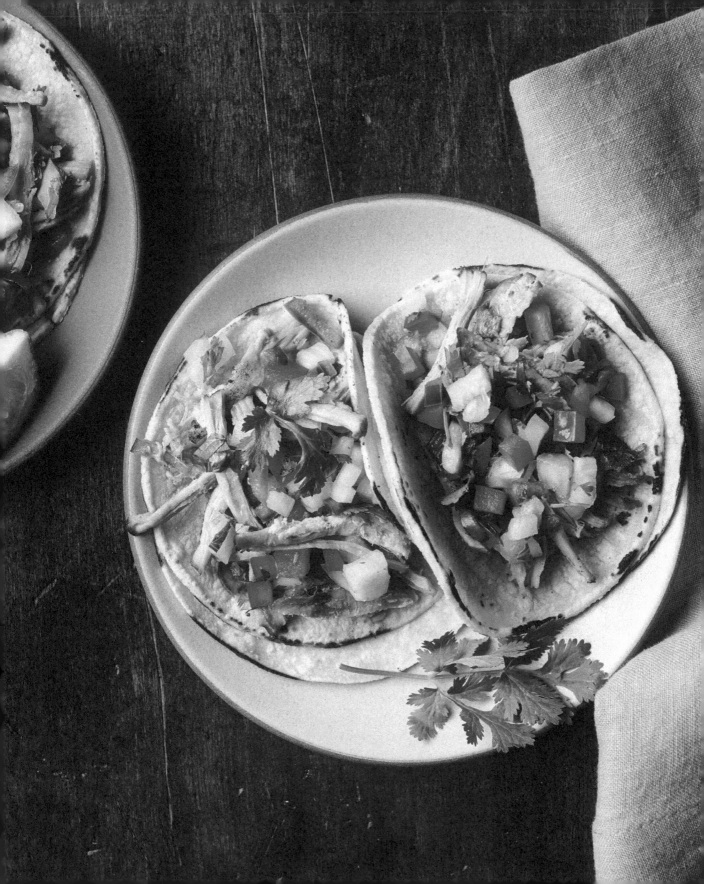

chapter 7
Beef and Pork

Korean Short Ribs . . . 122

Easy Chili . . . 123

Beef Stew . . . 124

French Onion Soup Dip Sandwiches . . . 126

Thai Red Curry Beef . . . 129

Kielbasa and Vegetable Stew . . . 131

Penne with Italian Sausage and Broccoli Rabe . . . 132

Mixed-Up Lasagna . . . 133

Char Siu . . . 134

Italian Pork Sandwiches . . . 136

Pork Tacos with Pineapple Salsa . . . 138

Ham and Potato Soup . . . 140

Korean Short Ribs

A little sweet, a bit tangy, and with a hint of spice, these short ribs hit all the right notes. Short ribs are a great cut for the Instant Pot®; for this recipe, buy English-style, not "flanken" cut, which require a different cooking time.

SERVES 2

PREP & FINISHING:
15 MINUTES

PRESSURE COOK:
40 MINUTES HIGH

RELEASE:
NATURAL
15 MINUTES,
THEN QUICK

TOTAL TIME:
1 HOUR 15 MINUTES,
PLUS 20 MINUTES
TO MARINATE

Per Serving
Calories: 1,110; Fat: 82 g;
Carbohydrates: 56 g;
Fiber: 4 g; Protein: 35 g;
Sodium: 2147 mg

2 pounds bone-in, English-style beef short ribs (about 4 large rib pieces)
½ teaspoon kosher salt
1 small onion, cut into chunks
1 small Asian or Bosc pear, peeled and cut into chunks
8 garlic cloves
1 tablespoon minced fresh ginger
¼ cup rice wine or dry sherry
⅓ cup soy sauce
2 teaspoons gochujang (Korean chile paste), Sriracha, or chili-garlic paste
3 tablespoons sugar
2 scallions, green part only, thinly sliced on the diagonal, for garnish

1. Sprinkle the short ribs on all sides with the salt. Place in a resealable plastic bag and let sit while you prepare the marinade.

2. For the marinade, place the onion and pear chunks in a blender jar. Add the garlic, ginger, rice wine, soy sauce, gochujang, and sugar. Pulse until the mixture is fairly smooth. (If you don't have a blender, grate the onion, apple, and garlic cloves and mix with the remaining ingredients.) Pour the marinade over the short ribs, manipulating the bag to make sure the meat is fully coated. Let them sit at room temperature for 20 minutes to an hour.

3. Place the ribs and marinade into the inner pot. Select Pressure Cook or Manual, and adjust the pressure to High and the time to 40 minutes. After cooking, let the pressure release naturally for 15 minutes, then quick release any remaining pressure.

4. Unlock the lid. Use tongs to remove the meat to a platter or shallow bowl. Spoon or blot off the fat from the surface of the liquid in the pot, or use a fat separator to remove it. If you like, simmer the sauce for a few minutes to thicken.

5. To serve, spoon some of the sauce over the ribs and sprinkle with the scallions.

Use It Up: If you have leftovers, cut the meat off the bones and add it to the Spicy Sesame Noodles and Vegetables (page 85).

Easy Chili

My go-to recipe for chili involves chunks of beef simmered for a few hours in an ancho chile sauce, with beans on the side. But I also enjoy the more typical combination of ground beef and beans with a chile and tomato sauce, and that's why I developed this version. If you can find "chili grind" beef, it gives a better texture to the chili, but regular ground beef works well. If you can't find ancho chile powder, you can substitute regular chili powder, but cut the oregano, salt, and cumin in half and adjust the seasoning after cooking.

1 tablespoon vegetable oil

1 pound coarse or regular ground beef

1 medium onion, chopped

1 medium jalapeño, chopped

1 large or 2 small garlic cloves, minced or pressed (about 2 teaspoons)

½ (14-ounce) can diced tomatoes

1 (14-ounce) can pinto beans, drained and rinsed

3 tablespoons ancho chile powder

1 teaspoon dried oregano

1½ teaspoons ground cumin

1 teaspoon kosher salt or ½ teaspoon fine salt

½ cup beef broth

SERVES 2

PREP & FINISHING:
10 MINUTES

SAUTÉ:
5 MINUTES

PRESSURE COOK:
12 MINUTES HIGH

RELEASE:
QUICK

TOTAL TIME:
35 MINUTES

Per Serving
Calories: 814; Fat: 52 g;
Carbohydrates: 46 g;
Fiber: 14 g; Protein: 41 g;
Sodium: 1718 mg

1. Select Sauté and adjust to High heat. Add the vegetable oil. When it's hot, add a big scoop of the beef. Press it into a disk and let it brown for 2 to 3 minutes without stirring. Add the onion and stir for a minute or so, getting up any browned bits of meat from the bottom of the pot. Add the remaining beef and stir to break it up.

2. Add the jalapeño, garlic, tomatoes, beans, chile powder, oregano, cumin, salt, and beef broth. Stir to combine.

3. Lock the lid into place. Select Pressure Cook or Manual, and adjust the pressure to High and the time to 12 minutes. After cooking, quick release the pressure. Taste and adjust the seasoning, if necessary.

4. If the chili is too thin, select Sauté and simmer until it thickens to your taste.

Use It Up: Use the other half of the tomatoes in Chicken Paprikash (page 112) or the Penne with Italian Sausage and Broccoli Rabe (page 132). If you have excess ground beef, use it in the Mixed-Up Lasagna (page 133).

Beef Stew

A generous amount of red wine makes this stew reminiscent of the classic beef bourguignon, but it's much less fussy. Cooking the beef and vegetables separately gives you meltingly tender beef with perfect vegetables—tender, but not falling apart.

SERVES 2

PREP & FINISHING:
10 MINUTES

SAUTE:
10 MINUTES

PRESSURE COOK:
20 MINUTES
HIGH *THEN*
4 MINUTES HIGH

RELEASE:
QUICK *THEN*
QUICK

TOTAL TIME:
55 MINUTES

Per Serving
Calories: 664; Fat: 25 g;
Carbohydrates: 35 g;
Fiber: 5 g; Protein: 58 g;
Sodium: 692 mg

1 pound boneless beef chuck roast, cut about 1½ inches thick
½ teaspoon kosher salt
2 tablespoons extra-virgin olive oil
¾ cup dry red wine
1 tablespoon all-purpose flour
1½ cups low-sodium beef stock
2 medium garlic cloves
1 small onion, quartered
1 bay leaf
¼ teaspoon freshly ground black pepper
8 ounces small red potatoes, quartered
2 medium carrots, cut into 1-inch pieces

1. Sprinkle the beef with the salt. Select Sauté and adjust to High heat. Add the olive oil to the inner pot and heat until it shimmers. Add the beef and brown it for 3 minutes, then turn and brown the other side. Remove the beef to a rack or plate and set aside to cool slightly.

2. Add the wine to the pot and stir, scraping the bottom of the pot to dissolve the browned bits. Bring to a boil and cook for 1 to 2 minutes, or until the wine has reduced by about a third.

3. While the wine reduces, cut the beef into pieces about 1-inch square.

4. In a small bowl, whisk together the flour and beef stock. Add it to the pot, along with the garlic cloves, onion quarters, and bay leaf. Add the beef cubes with any accumulated juices.

5. Lock the lid in place. Select Manual, and adjust the pressure to High and the time to 20 minutes. After cooking, quick release the pressure. Unlock the lid. Fish out the onion quarters, garlic cloves (if they haven't dissolved), and bay leaf.

6. Add the pepper, potatoes, and carrots. Lock the lid in place. Select Manual, and adjust the pressure to High and the time to 4 minutes. After cooking, quick release the pressure.

7. Unlock the lid. If you want a thicker sauce, select Sauté and adjust to Medium heat. Bring to a simmer until the sauce reaches the texture you desire.

Double It: If you want to make extra stew for freezing, double the ingredients, but cook only through step 5. To serve, defrost the stew and bring to a simmer on the Sauté setting. Add the potatoes and carrots and finish steps 6 and 7 (potatoes tend to get mushy when frozen).

Make It Gluten-Free: Omit the flour. If desired, after cooking mix 1 tablespoon cornstarch with 1 tablespoon water and add to the sauce. Bring to a simmer to thicken the stew.

Mini Modification: You may have to sear the beef in two batches, which will increase the prep and total time.

French Onion Soup Dip Sandwiches

Think of this recipe as a cross between a French dip sandwich and French onion soup. I got the idea for it when I had some French onion soup in the refrigerator and also some cooked leftover steak. There wasn't enough soup for a whole serving, but I figured it would make a perfect jus substitute for a French dip sandwich. I had some Gruyère, so that went on as well. It turned out so well that I decided to make it into a real recipe. You probably won't need the whole 2 pounds of beef for two sandwiches, but it can be difficult to find a smaller piece of chuck. The leftovers keep well for several days.

SERVES 2

PREP & FINISHING:
10 MINUTES

SAUTÉ:
8 MINUTES

PRESSURE COOK:
35 MINUTES HIGH

RELEASE:
NATURAL
8 MINUTES,
THEN QUICK

TOTAL TIME:
1 HOUR

Per Serving
Calories: 983; Fat: 45 g;
Carbohydrates: 68 g;
Fiber: 12 g; Protein: 77 g;
Sodium: 806 mg

2 pounds chuck roast, cut about 2 inches thick

1 teaspoon kosher salt, divided

2 tablespoons extra-virgin olive oil

4 cups (about 1 pound) sliced onion

⅓ cup dry sherry

¾ cup low-sodium beef broth

½ teaspoon anchovy paste or 1 teaspoon Marmite (optional)

2 teaspoons Worcestershire sauce

1 teaspoon dried thyme or 1 fresh thyme sprig

2 hoagie or sub rolls

4 ounces Gruyère or other Swiss-style cheese, grated

1. Sprinkle the beef on all sides with ½ teaspoon of salt.

2. Select Sauté and adjust to Medium heat. Add the olive oil to the inner pot and heat until it shimmers. Add the beef. Cook without turning for 3 minutes, or until browned. Turn and brown the other side. Remove the beef to a plate or sheet pan.

3. Add the onion to the fat in the pot. Sprinkle with ¼ teaspoon of salt and stir until they soften and begin to turn light brown. Pour the sherry into the pot. Scrape up the browned bits from the bottom of the pot and cook until it has reduced by about half. Add the broth and stir to get up any remaining browned bits from the bottom of the pot. Stir in the anchovy paste or Marmite (if using), Worcestershire sauce, thyme, and the remaining ¼ teaspoon of salt.

4. Lock the lid in place. Select Pressure Cook or Manual, and adjust the pressure to High and the time to 35 minutes. After cooking, let the pressure release naturally for 8 minutes, then quick release any remaining pressure.

5. Unlock the lid. Use tongs to remove the meat to a cutting board. Let it cool and then cut into chunks or shred it.

6. Degrease the sauce. If you have one, strain the liquid into a fat separator, saving the onion. When the fat has separated, pour the sauce back into the pot. If you don't have a separator, after removing the meat, let the sauce cool until any fat has risen to the top. Remove as much fat as possible with a spoon or use paper towels to blot it off.

7. While the sauce is separating, prepare the rolls. Preheat the broiler. Split the rolls almost through and, if desired, remove some of the soft bread from the interior. Place on a baking sheet. Carefully spread the rolls apart without separating the two halves and sprinkle the cheese over both sides of the bread. Place under the broiler until the cheese is melted and just starting to brown.

8. Return the reserved onions to the pot. Taste the broth and add more salt if necessary. Return the meat to the sauce. While the rolls toast, select Sauté and adjust to Medium heat. Bring the sauce and meat to a simmer.

9. To serve, pile some meat and onions on each roll and close the sandwich. Slice in half, if desired. Pour the sauce into two bowls and serve with the sandwiches for dipping.

Make It New: Slice the extra beef and serve with a little of the sauce. German Potato Salad (page 40) or Smashed Red Potatoes with Bacon (page 48) are excellent sides.

Mini Modification: You may have to sear the beef in two batches, which will increase the prep and total time.

Use It Up: Use extra anchovy paste in the Broccoli Rabe with Lemon-Anchovy Vinaigrette (page 52).

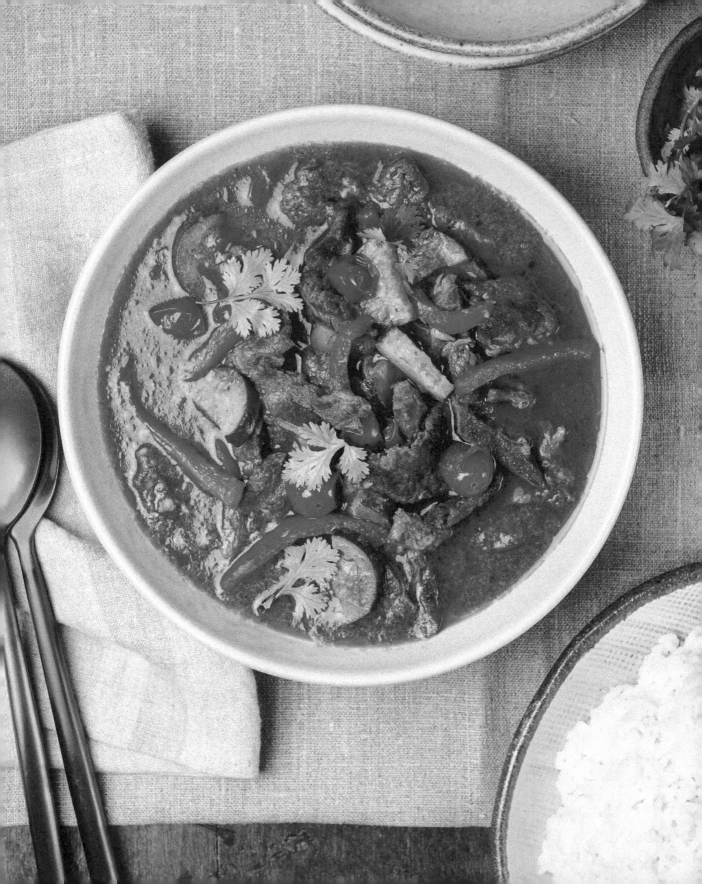

Thai Red Curry Beef

I have friends who make their own Thai curry pastes. I admire them, but it's just too much work for me. I use Mae Ploy brand paste, and am pleased with the results. This curry cooks while the rice steams, giving you a complete dinner in one pot. Blade roast is a cut of shoulder (a flat-iron steak is half a blade roast) that's more tender than chuck roast, but if you can't find it, just use regular chuck, sliced thin.

1 (14-ounce) can coconut milk

1 ounce Thai red curry paste (about 2 tablespoons)

12 ounces blade roast or flat-iron steak, cut into ¼-inch-thick slices

½ small onion, sliced

½ cup long-grain white rice, rinsed

½ cup plus 1 tablespoon water

¼ teaspoon kosher salt

½ medium zucchini, cut into ¼-inch rounds then cut into half moons

½ medium red bell pepper, seeded and cut into 1-inch pieces

½ pint cherry tomatoes, halved

2 tablespoons coarsely chopped fresh basil or cilantro

½ teaspoon freshly squeezed lime juice (optional)

½ teaspoon sugar (optional)

¼ teaspoon fish sauce or soy sauce (optional)

SERVES 2

PREP & FINISHING:
10 MINUTES

SAUTÉ:
6 MINUTES

PRESSURE COOK:
7 MINUTES HIGH

RELEASE:
NATURAL 10 MINUTES, THEN QUICK

TOTAL TIME:
45 MINUTES

Per Serving
Calories: 945; Fat: 61 g; Carbohydrates: 59 g; Fiber: 7 g; Protein: 45 g; Sodium: 690 mg

1. Pour the coconut milk into the inner pot. Add the curry paste and stir to combine. Add the beef and onion.

2. Place a trivet in the pot that's tall enough to clear the meat.

3. Place the rice in a heat-proof bowl that holds at least 3 cups. Add the water and salt, and stir to dissolve the salt. Place the bowl on top of the trivet.

4. Lock the lid into place. Select Pressure Cook or Manual, and adjust the pressure to High and the time to 7 minutes.

5. While the beef and rice cook, chop the vegetables.

6. After cooking, let the pressure release naturally for 10 minutes, then quick release any remaining pressure. ➤

7. Unlock the lid. Carefully remove the rice bowl and trivet. Fluff the rice with a fork and cover with aluminum foil. Set aside.

8. Select Sauté and adjust to Medium heat. Add the zucchini, bell pepper, and tomatoes and bring to a simmer. Cook, stirring occasionally, for 5 to 6 minutes, or until the vegetables are tender. Stir in the basil. Taste and adjust the seasoning as needed with lime juice, sugar, or fish sauce (if using).

9. To serve, divide the rice between two bowls and top with the curry. You may not need all the sauce.

Use It Up: Use the other half of the zucchini in Minestrone (page 74). Use the remaining tomatoes in Farfalle with Salmon, Fennel, and Tomatoes (page 92). Use the rest of the bell pepper in Spicy Chicken Lettuce Cups (page 108) or the Southwestern Black Bean Salad (page 60).

Kielbasa and Vegetable Stew

Maybe it's the German side of my heritage, but whatever the reason, I love smoked sausages like kielbasa. This easy one-pot meal adds vegetables and a robust broth to the sausage for a quick weeknight dinner.

10 ounces kielbasa, Polish sausage, or other smoked sausage, cut into 1½-inch pieces

1 small onion, cut into 8 wedges

2 garlic cloves, minced or pressed

1 large or 2 medium carrots, cut into 1-inch pieces (or ⅔ cup baby carrots)

8 ounces (2-inch) red potatoes, quartered

2 cups roughly chopped white cabbage

½ teaspoon kosher salt

1 cup Chicken Stock (page 158)

¼ teaspoon freshly ground black pepper

½ teaspoon caraway seeds

½ teaspoon smoked or regular paprika

½ teaspoon dried thyme

2 tablespoons whole-grain mustard

¼ cup chopped fresh parsley

SERVES 2

PREP & FINISHING:
10 MINUTES

PRESSURE COOK:
4 MINUTES HIGH

RELEASE:
QUICK

TOTAL TIME:
25 MINUTES

Per Serving
Calories: 487; Fat: 16 g;
Carbohydrates: 38 g;
Fiber: 7 g; Protein: 50 g;
Sodium: 1454 mg

1. In the inner pot, add the sausage, onion, garlic, carrots, potatoes, and cabbage, and stir gently.

2. In a medium bowl, stir together the salt, chicken stock, pepper, caraway seeds, paprika, thyme, and mustard. Pour this over the sausage and vegetables.

3. Lock the lid into place. Select Pressure Cook or Manual, and adjust the pressure to High and the time to 4 minutes. After cooking, quick release the pressure.

4. Unlock the lid. Stir in the parsley. Test a carrot or potato; if they aren't soft enough for your taste, simmer the stew for a couple of minutes.

Double It: If you have a 6-quart Instant Pot®, you can easily double this recipe, but the greater volume of liquid will cause the pot to take longer to come to pressure, so reduce the cook time to 3 minutes. It's not recommended to double the recipe if you're using the Mini.

Use It Up: Use the rest of the cabbage in the slaw for the Barbecue Chicken Sandwiches with Slaw (page 116).

Penne with Italian Sausage and Broccoli Rabe

Sometimes I think there's nothing better than pasta with Italian sausage. It's so easy, so delicious, and so comforting. Broccoli rabe not only adds a contrasting flavor and texture, but its addition means you don't have to worry about vegetables on the side. Garlic bread is all you need to finish the meal.

SERVES 2

PREP & FINISHING:
10 MINUTES

SAUTÉ:
5 MINUTES

PRESSURE COOK:
0 MINUTES HIGH, PLUS
6 MINUTES HIGH

RELEASE:
QUICK

TOTAL TIME:
40 MINUTES

Per Serving
Calories: 911; Fat: 62 g;
Carbohydrates: 56 g;
Fiber: 10 g; Protein: 32 g;
Sodium: 1067 mg

2 tablespoons extra-virgin olive oil

½ pound hot or sweet Italian sausage, casings removed and cut into 1-inch pieces

½ small onion, chopped (about ¼ cup)

¼ cup white wine

½ (14-ounce) can diced tomatoes

½ teaspoon kosher salt, divided

4 ounces penne pasta

1¼ cups water

¼ cup heavy (whipping) cream

4 ounces steamed broccoli rabe (see page 52)

1. Select Sauté and adjust to Medium heat. Add the olive oil to the inner pot and heat until it shimmers. Add the sausage in a single layer. Brown the sausage pieces on all sides, then push them to the sides of the pot. Add the onion, and cook, stirring often, until the onion pieces separate and begin to soften, about 2 minutes. Add the wine and stir, scraping the bottom of the pot to dissolve the browned bits. Pour in the tomatoes, salt, pasta, and water. Stir to combine.

2. Lock the lid in place. Select Pressure Cook or Manual, and adjust the pressure to High and the time to 6 minutes. After cooking, quick release the pressure.

3. Unlock the lid. Test the pasta; it should be tender with just a slightly firm center. Stir in the cream and broccoli rabe, and bring to a simmer to heat through. Adjust the seasoning, if necessary, and serve.

Make It Dairy-Free: The pasta is delicious without the cream; add a tablespoon or so of olive oil after cooking, if desired.

Use It Up: If you have a whole bunch of broccoli rabe, it's easy to steam it all, then use the remainder in the White Bean Stew with Broccoli Rabe (page 56) or Italian Pork Sandwiches (page 136). If you have leftover Italian sausage, you can use it instead of ground beef in the Mixed-Up Lasagna (page 133).

Mixed-Up Lasagna

I'm really picky when it comes to lasagna. It's got to contain fresh pasta, home-made tomato sauce, and balsamella sauce, which means it's time consuming and reserved for special occasions. When I feel like the flavors of lasagna but I want them fast, I turn to this dish. Even though it isn't really lasagna at all, it satisfies my craving with a fraction of the work and without the mess.

½ pound ground beef or Italian sausage (or a combination)

1 cup water

4 ounces farfalle pasta

12 ounces Marinara Sauce (page 160)

¼ teaspoon kosher salt

2 ounces ricotta cheese, at room temperature (about ⅓ cup)

2 teaspoons chopped fresh parsley

¼ teaspoon freshly ground black pepper

¾ cup loosely packed shredded mozzarella cheese (about 2 ounces)

¼ cup grated Parmesan cheese

SERVES 2

PREP & FINISHING:
10 MINUTES

SAUTÉ:
5 MINUTES

PRESSURE COOK:
6 MINUTES HIGH

RELEASE:
QUICK

TOTAL TIME:
35 MINUTES

Per Serving
Calories: 768; Fat: 46 g;
Carbohydrates: 53 g;
Fiber: 4 g; Protein: 36 g;
Sodium: 1508 mg

1. Select Sauté and adjust to High heat. Add the beef to the inner pot and let it brown, without stirring, for 2 to 3 minutes. When one side is browned, stir the beef to break it up. Cancel Sauté.

2. Pour in the water and scrape up any browned bits from the bottom. Add the pasta, marinara sauce, and salt. Stir to combine.

3. Lock the lid into place. Select Pressure Cook or Manual, and adjust the pressure to High and the time to 6 minutes.

4. While the pasta cooks, in a small bowl, mix the ricotta, parsley, and pepper.

5. After cooking, quick release the pressure.

6. Unlock the lid. Test the pasta; it should be tender with just a slightly firm center. Stir in the mozzarella, just until melted.

7. To serve, ladle the pasta into two bowls and top with a scoop of the ricotta mixture. Sprinkle the Parmesan over top.

Mini Modification: In step 3, cut the cooking time to 5 minutes.

Use It Up: Use leftover ricotta cheese in the Ricotta Cheesecakes with Balsamic Strawberries (page 152) or the Savory Ham and Cheese Egg Cups (page 35).

Char Siu

If you've ever wandered through the Chinatown area of a big city, chances are you've seen shops with big strips of red-tinted barbecue pork hanging in the windows. Crisp and sticky on the outside and tender on the inside, it's one of my favorite Chinese dishes. My version isn't barbecued, but it's faster and easier than the traditional method, and it's still delicious. The liquid smoke is optional, but it does help mimic the flavor of the barbecue.

SERVES 2

PREP & FINISHING:
13 MINUTES

PRESSURE COOK:
18 MINUTES HIGH

RELEASE:
QUICK

TOTAL TIME:
45 MINUTES,
PLUS 1 HOUR
TO MARINATE

Per Serving
Calories: 661; Fat: 42 g;
Carbohydrates: 39 g;
Fiber: 1 g; Protein: 33 g;
Sodium: 1346 mg

1¼ pounds boneless shoulder country ribs
1 tablespoon sugar
2 tablespoons honey
¼ cup hoisin sauce
3 tablespoons soy sauce
1 teaspoon Chinese five-spice powder
1 teaspoon liquid smoke (optional)
2 tablespoons Chicken Stock (page 158) or store bought (low-sodium)
1 tablespoon vegetable or coconut oil

1. Place the ribs in a heavy resealable plastic bag.

2. In a small bowl, whisk together the sugar, honey, hoisin sauce, soy sauce, five-spice powder, liquid smoke (if using), stock, and oil. Pour it over the ribs and seal the bag. Manipulate the bag to coat the ribs in the sauce. Let the pork marinate at least 20 minutes to 1 hour, or overnight in the refrigerator.

3. Place the ribs and marinade in the inner pot. Select Pressure Cook or Manual, and adjust the pressure to High and the time to 18 minutes.

4. While the pork cooks, preheat the broiler. Place a rack in a baking pan or on a baking sheet.

5. After cooking, quick release the pressure.

6. Unlock the lid. Use tongs to remove the ribs to the rack. Select Sauté and adjust to High heat. Boil the sauce for 5 minutes, or until thickened somewhat (like barbecue sauce).

7. Baste the ribs with some of the marinade and place them under the broiler. Broil until crisp and browned, 3 to 5 minutes. Turn and baste with more sauce and broil for another few minutes.

8. Slice and serve.

Double It: You can double the entire recipe and freeze half of it (with marinade), or cook twice the amount of meat in a single batch of marinade.

Make It A Meal: This goes well with the Rice Pilaf with Bacon and Water Chestnuts (page 64), or serve it with Basic White or Brown Rice (page 163) and the Warm Thai-Style Green Bean and Tomato Salad (page 50).

Italian Pork Sandwiches

The ingredients in this sandwich, which hails from Philadelphia, might seem like an odd combination, but the slight bitterness of the broccoli rabe is a great foil for the rich pork and tangy cheese. The recipe takes some time and effort, but I think it's worth it. If you don't have all the herbs and spices, don't worry—just use what you have.

SERVES 2

PREP & FINISHING:
15 MINUTES

SAUTÉ:
8 MINUTES

PRESSURE COOK:
25 MINUTES HIGH

RELEASE:
NATURAL
10 MINUTES,
THEN QUICK

TOTAL TIME:
1 HOUR

Per Serving
Calories: 916; Fat: 56 g;
Carbohydrates: 47 g;
Fiber: 11 g; Protein: 42 g;
Sodium: 1153 mg

1 pound bone-in (or ¾ pound boneless) pork country shoulder ribs
¾ teaspoon kosher salt, divided
2 tablespoons extra-virgin olive oil
1 small onion, thinly sliced
3 garlic cloves, minced
½ cup red wine
¼ cup Chicken Stock (page 158) or store bought (low-sodium)
1 teaspoon fennel seeds
1 teaspoon dried thyme

1 bay leaf
½ teaspoon red pepper flakes
¼ teaspoon freshly ground black pepper
1 fresh rosemary sprig
1 fresh parsley sprig
4 ounces steamed Broccoli Rabe (see page 52), trimmed and cut into 1- or 2-inch pieces
2 hoagie or sub rolls
3 ounces provolone cheese (mild or sharp or a combination), grated

1. Sprinkle ½ teaspoon of salt on all sides of the country ribs.

2. Select Sauté and adjust to Medium heat. Add the olive oil to the pot and heat until it shimmers. Add the ribs. Cook without turning for 3 minutes, or until browned on one side. Turn and brown the other side. Remove the ribs to a plate or baking sheet.

3. Add the onion to the fat in the pot. Sprinkle with ¼ teaspoon of salt and stir until the onion pieces soften and begin to turn light brown, about 2 minutes. Add the garlic and stir.

4. Pour the wine into the pot. Scrape up the browned bits from the bottom of the pot and cook until the wine has reduced by about half. Add the stock and stir to get up any remaining browned bits. Add the fennel seeds, thyme, bay leaf, red pepper flakes, pepper, rosemary sprig, and parsley sprig. Stir to distribute. Return the meat pieces to the pot.

5. Lock the lid in place. Select Pressure Cook or Manual, and adjust the pressure to High and the time to 25 minutes. After cooking, let the pressure release naturally for 10 minutes, then quick release any remaining pressure.

6. Unlock the lid. Use tongs to remove the meat to a cutting board. Let it cool and then cut into chunks or shred it.

7. Degrease the sauce. If you have one, strain the liquid into a fat separator, saving the solids (the onions, garlic, and spices). When the fat has separated, pour the sauce back into the pot. If you don't have a separator, after removing the meat, let the sauce cool until any fat has risen to the top. Remove as much fat as possible with a spoon or use paper towels to blot it off.

8. Return the reserved solids from the sauce to the pot, removing and discarding the bay leaf and herb stems. If the sauce is too thin, select Sauté and adjust to Medium heat. Bring to a boil and reduce until thickened slightly. Taste and add more salt, if necessary. Return the meat to the sauce. Add the broccoli rabe to warm it up.

9. To serve, split the rolls almost through and, if desired, remove some of the soft bread from the interior. Carefully spread the rolls apart without separating the two halves and sprinkle the cheese over both sides of the bread. Top with the warm meat and broccoli rabe and drizzle with some sauce.

Double It: You can double the meat without doubling the sauce.

Make It New: Serve the extra pork on another night with Crispy Salt and Vinegar Potatoes (page 38) or Roasted Sweet Potatoes and Beets with Rosemary (page 46).

Mini Modification: You may have to sear the pork in two batches, which will increase the prep and total time.

Use It Up: If you have a whole bunch of broccoli rabe, it's easy to steam it all, then use the remainder in the White Bean Stew with Broccoli Rabe (page 56) or Penne with Italian Sausage and Broccoli Rabe (page 132).

Pork Tacos with Pineapple Salsa

More complex than carnitas, the meat for these tacos is loosely based on cochinita pibil, *or seasoned pork roasted in a pit in the ground. Lacking a pit in the backyard (actually, lacking a backyard of any kind), I've come up with this recipe, which provides the same flavors and is much easier. I like to pair the mildly spicy meat with pineapple salsa, but you can use whatever salsa you prefer.*

SERVES 2

PREP & FINISHING:
10 MINUTES

PRESSURE COOK:
25 MINUTES HIGH

RELEASE:
NATURAL
10 MINUTES,
THEN QUICK

TOTAL TIME:
50 MINUTES

Per Serving
Calories: 558; Fat: 20 g;
Carbohydrates: 39 g;
Fiber: 5 g; Protein: 57 g;
Sodium: 997 mg

1 teaspoon kosher salt

½ teaspoon dried oregano

¼ teaspoon ground cumin

Pinch cinnamon

1 tablespoon extra-virgin olive oil

¼ teaspoon freshly ground black pepper

1 teaspoon liquid smoke (optional)

2 tablespoons freshly squeezed orange juice

1½ pounds country ribs, or pork shoulder cut into 2-inch strips

4 garlic cloves, pressed

¼ cup freshly squeezed lime juice

4 or 6 small corn or flour tortillas, warmed

For the salsa

4 ounces fresh pineapple, trimmed and chopped (about ½ cup)

¼ small red bell pepper, seeded and chopped

¼ small onion, chopped (about 2 tablespoons)

1 small serrano pepper or jalapeño, seeded and chopped

2 tablespoons chopped cilantro

1 to 2 teaspoons freshly squeezed lime juice

¼ teaspoon kosher salt, or more as needed

1. In a small bowl, mix the salt, oregano, cumin, cinnamon, olive oil, pepper, liquid smoke (if using), and orange juice. Sprinkle over the country ribs and lightly rub the spices into the meat. If you have time, let the ribs rest for 30 minutes (or up to overnight in the refrigerator).

2. Add the garlic and lime juice to the inner pot. Place the ribs in the pot, arranging them in a single layer. Lock the lid into place. Select Manual or Pressure Cook; adjust the pressure to High and the time to 25 minutes.

3. While the pork is cooking, make the salsa. In a medium bowl, mix the pineapple, bell pepper, onion, pepper, cilantro, 1 teaspoon of lime juice, and salt. Taste and add the second teaspoon of lime juice if you want it more tart.

4. After cooking, let the pressure release naturally for 10 minutes, then quick release any remaining pressure.

5. Unlock the lid. Use tongs to remove the ribs to a plate or cutting board. Use forks or your hands to shred the meat into bite-sized chunks, discarding any fat or gristle. To serve, spoon ¼ cup or so of pork onto a tortilla and top with a spoonful of salsa.

Double It: The meat doubles easily and makes great leftovers. Double the ingredients and leave the cooking time the same. The salsa can be doubled but doesn't keep for more than a day or so refrigerated.

Use It Up: Use extra pineapple in Sweet and Sour Chicken (page 114). Use the rest of the red bell pepper in Spicy Chicken Lettuce Cups (page 108) or Thai Red Curry Beef (page 129).

Ham and Potato Soup

For me, it's always a toss-up with potato soup: Do I prefer the potatoes in chunks, or mashed up into the broth for a thicker soup? I've finally decided I can have it both ways. In this hearty soup, red potatoes are steamed separately and added at the end to preserve their shape, while a russet gets mashed into the soup for thickening.

SERVES 2

PREP & FINISHING:
10 MINUTES

SAUTÉ:
5 MINUTES

PRESSURE COOK:
3 MINUTES HIGH,
PLUS 7 MINUTES
HIGH

RELEASE:
QUICK *THEN* NATURAL
8 MINUTES,
THEN QUICK

TOTAL TIME:
45 MINUTES

Per Serving
Calories: 670; Fat: 29 g;
Carbohydrates: 82 g;
Fiber: 10 g; Protein: 24 g;
Sodium: 1159 mg

6 ounces (about 3) small red potatoes, cut into ½-inch pieces
2 tablespoons unsalted butter
½ small onion, chopped
1 carrot, chopped
1 tablespoon all-purpose flour
1 teaspoon mustard powder
1½ cups low-sodium chicken stock
1 small (about 8 ounces) russet potato, peeled and cut into 1-inch cubes

½ teaspoon kosher salt
½ teaspoon freshly ground black pepper
1 teaspoon Worcestershire sauce
1 bay leaf
¾ cup diced ham
½ cup half-and-half, or ¼ cup heavy (whipping) cream and ¼ cup milk
¼ cup shredded Cheddar cheese
1 scallion, green part only, chopped, for garnish

1. Pour 1 cup of water into the inner pot. Arrange the red potatoes as evenly as possible in a steaming basket and place the basket in the pot. Lock the lid into place. Select Steam and adjust the pressure to High and the time to 3 minutes. After cooking, quick release the pressure. Unlock the lid, remove the basket, and set the potatoes aside. Empty the pot and return it to the base.

2. Select Sauté and adjust to Medium heat. Add the butter. When it has stopped foaming, add the onion and carrot and cook, stirring often, for 2 minutes or until the onion pieces have separated and begun to soften. Add the flour and mustard powder, and stir to coat the onions. Cook, stirring, for 2 minutes, or until the flour has darkened slightly in color. Add the stock and stir, scraping up any bits stuck to the bottom of the pot. Add the russet potato, salt, pepper, Worcestershire sauce, and bay leaf. Stir to combine.

3. Lock the lid into place. Select Pressure Cook or Manual, and adjust the pressure to High and the time to 7 minutes. After cooking, let the pressure release naturally for 8 minutes, then quick release any remaining pressure.

4. Unlock the lid. Use a potato masher to break up the potato chunks and thicken the soup. Stir in the ham, red potatoes, and half-and-half. Select Sauté and adjust to Low heat. Bring to a simmer until the potatoes and ham are warmed through.

5. Serve garnished with the cheese and scallion.

Double It: Double the ingredients and leave the cooking time the same.

Time Saver: You can skip the initial steaming of the red potatoes if you want to save time. Cut them slightly larger and cook with the soup. They may fall apart a bit, but that's okay.

Use It Up: Use leftover ham in the Savory Ham and Cheese Egg Cups (page 35).

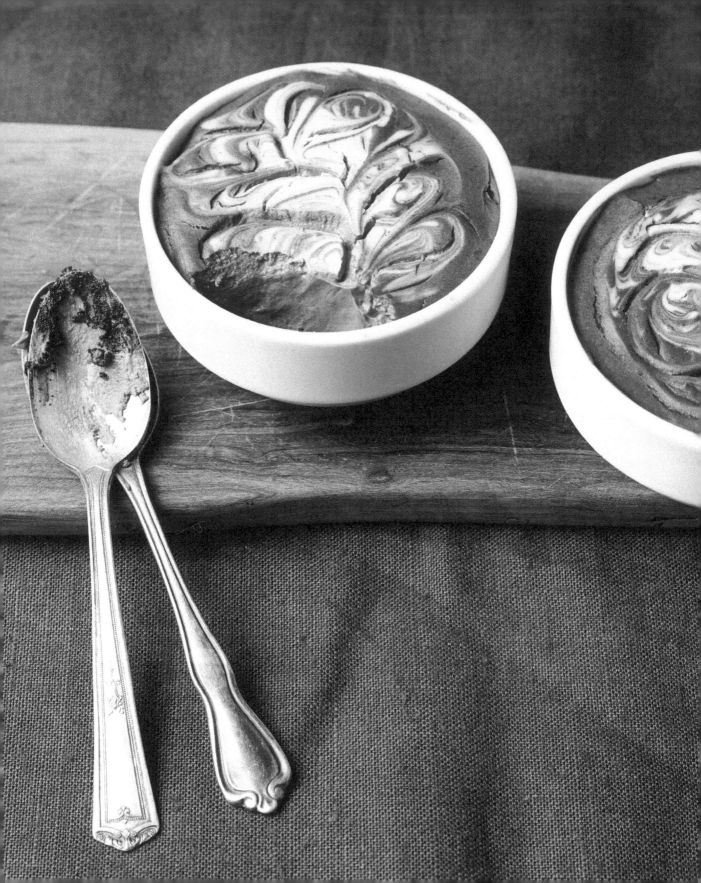

chapter 8
Desserts

Maple Nutmeg Custard . . . 144

Citrus Custard . . . 145

Spiced Peach Bread Pudding . . . 146

Coconut-Vanilla Rice Pudding . . . 147

Lemon Mousse . . . 148

Mini Chocolate Marble Cheesecakes . . . 150

Ricotta Cheesecakes with Balsamic Strawberries . . . 152

Carrot Cake . . . 154

Mini Chocolate Marble Cheesecakes, page 150

Maple Nutmeg Custard

Last year for Thanksgiving, I went in search of a new dessert. I found a recipe for a nutmeg and maple cream pie from The New York Times, *which turned out great. Streamlined and cut down, it makes a delicious custard for two. One caveat: It's crucial to use fresh nutmeg for this recipe. Once grated, nutmeg loses its aroma and flavor quickly.*

SERVES 2

PREP & FINISHING:
15 MINUTES

PRESSURE COOK:
8 MINUTES HIGH

RELEASE:
NATURAL
10 MINUTES,
THEN QUICK

TOTAL TIME:
45 MINUTES
PLUS 20 MINUTES
TO COOL
AND 2 HOURS
TO CHILL

Per Serving
Calories: 662; Fat: 51 g;
Carbohydrates: 35 g;
Fiber: 0 g; Protein: 8 g;
Sodium: 167 mg

1 cup heavy (whipping) cream
2 egg yolks
1 whole egg
¼ cup maple syrup
1 tablespoon brown sugar
Pinch kosher salt
½ teaspoon freshly grated nutmeg
½ teaspoon vanilla extract

1. In a medium bowl, whisk together the cream, egg yolks, and whole egg until thoroughly combined. Whisk in the maple syrup, brown sugar, salt, nutmeg, and vanilla. Pour into two (1½-cup) ramekins or custard cups.

2. Add 1 cup of water to the inner pot. Place a trivet in the pot and then place the ramekins on top. Cover the ramekins with a piece of aluminum foil to keep condensation off the top of the custards. Lock the lid into place. Select Pressure Cook or Manual, and adjust the pressure to High and the time to 8 minutes. When cooking is complete, let the pressure release naturally for 10 minutes, then quick release any remaining pressure.

3. Unlock the lid. Carefully remove the foil, and use tongs to remove the ramekins from the pot. Let cool at room temperature for 20 minutes or so, then refrigerate until chilled, about 2 hours.

Double It: Use four ramekins to make a double batch of this custard. Depending on the size of your ramekins, you may need to stack them, or cook in two batches (if you have a Mini). If cooking in two batches, empty the water, let the inner pot cool, and use a fresh cup of water for steaming.

Citrus Custard

This is another pie recipe cut down and turned into a custard for two—this one based on a recipe from Epicurious. You can serve it with whipped cream for a fancier version, but I'm such a citrus fan that I like it plain. If you like a sweeter dessert, add an extra tablespoon or two of sugar.

2 large eggs

½ cup sugar

1 teaspoon finely grated
orange zest

½ teaspoon finely grated
lemon zest

¼ cup freshly squeezed
orange juice

¼ cup freshly squeezed
lemon juice

2 tablespoons heavy
(whipping) cream

1. In a small bowl, whisk together the eggs and sugar. Add the orange zest, lemon zest, orange juice, lemon juice, and cream, and whisk until smooth. Pour into two (1½-cup) ramekins or custard cups.

2. Add 1 cup of water to the inner pot. Place a trivet in the pot and then place the ramekins on top. Cover the ramekins with a piece of aluminum foil to keep condensation off the top of the custards. Lock the lid into place. Select Pressure Cook or Manual, and adjust the pressure to Low and the time to 6 minutes. After cooking, let the pressure release naturally for 10 minutes, then quick release any remaining pressure.

3. Unlock the lid. Carefully remove the foil, and use tongs to remove the ramekins from the pot. Let cool at room temperature for 20 minutes or so, then refrigerate until chilled, about 2 hours.

Double It: Use four ramekins to make a double batch of this custard. Depending on the size of your ramekins, you may need to stack them, or cook in two batches (if you have a Mini). If cooking in two batches, empty the water, let the inner pot cool, and use a fresh cup of water for steaming.

Lux Modification: In step 2, keep the cooking time the same, but quick release the pressure after 7 minutes.

Use It Up: If you have part of an orange left, you can save it and use the juice in the Carrot Cake (page 154), Curried Cauliflower Soup (page 76), or Pork Tacos with Pineapple Salsa (page 138).

SERVES 2

PREP & FINISHING:
10 MINUTES

PRESSURE COOK:
6 MINUTES LOW

RELEASE:
NATURAL 10 MINUTES,
THEN QUICK

TOTAL TIME:
35 MINUTES, PLUS
20 MINUTES TO COOL
AND 2 HOURS TO CHILL

Per Serving
Calories: 333; Fat: 11 g;
Carbohydrates: 55 g;
Fiber: 0 g; Protein: 7 g;
Sodium: 82 mg

Spiced Peach Bread Pudding

When you develop recipes for a living as I do, you come across combinations of flavors and ingredients that you turn to over and over. For me, the duo of cinnamon and cardamom is one such combination. It's especially great with stone fruit like peaches. But if you don't like those spices, ginger or fresh grated nutmeg can stand in.

SERVES 2

PREP & FINISHING:
10 MINUTES

PRESSURE COOK:
10 MINUTES HIGH

RELEASE:
QUICK

TOTAL TIME:
30 MINUTES,
PLUS 10 MINUTES
TO COOL

Per Serving
Calories: 310; Fat: 19 g;
Carbohydrates: 29 g;
Fiber: 1 g; Protein: 8 g;
Sodium: 337 mg

1 tablespoon unsalted
    butter, melted
3 teaspoons brown
    sugar, divided
1 large egg
⅔ cup whole milk
¼ teaspoon vanilla extract
Pinch kosher salt

½ teaspoon cinnamon
¼ teaspoon cardamom, ginger,
    or nutmeg
2 cups (¾-inch) pound
    cake cubes
¼ cup chopped frozen
    peaches, thawed

1. In two (1-cup) custard cups or ramekins, brush the insides (bottom and sides) with the melted butter. Sprinkle ½ teaspoon of brown sugar on the bottom of each cup.

2. In a small bowl, whisk together the egg, milk, vanilla, salt, cinnamon, cardamom, and the remaining 2 teaspoons of brown sugar. Add the pound cake cubes and toss to coat with the egg mixture. Let the cake soak in the egg mixture for 2 to 3 minutes, gently tossing several times so the mixture is evenly distributed. Stir in the peaches.

3. When the egg mixture has mostly soaked into the cake cubes, divide the mixture between the two cups.

4. Add 1 cup of water to the inner pot. Place a trivet in the pot and then place the ramekins on top. Cover the ramekins with a piece of aluminum foil to keep condensation off the top of the puddings. Lock the lid into place. Select Pressure Cook or Manual, and adjust the pressure to High and the time to 10 minutes. After cooking, quick release the pressure.

5. Unlock the lid. Carefully remove the foil, and use tongs to remove the ramekins from the pot. Let cool at room temperature for 10 minutes or so. Serve warm, plain or with whipped cream or vanilla ice cream.

Coconut-Vanilla Rice Pudding

This dairy-free, gluten-free dessert is rich and creamy—comfort food at its best. Adding the vanilla after cooking lets the flavor and aroma shine through. For an extra-rich pudding, scrape a tablespoon or so of the coconut fat from the coconut milk and stir it in after cooking.

⅓ cup arborio rice

1 cup coconut milk

2 tablespoons sugar

Pinch kosher salt

½ teaspoon vanilla

1 tablespoon coconut fat from the milk (optional)

1. Add the rice to the inner pot. Add the coconut milk, sugar, and salt, and stir to dissolve the sugar.

2. Lock the lid into place. Select Pressure Cook or Manual, and adjust the pressure to High and the time to 20 minutes. After cooking, let the pressure release naturally for 10 minutes, then quick release any remaining pressure.

3. Unlock the lid. Stir in the vanilla and coconut fat (if using). Stir the rice pudding thoroughly until the dessert is creamy. Serve warm or chill and serve cold.

Double It: Double all ingredients; keep the cooking time the same.

Use It Up: Extra rice can be used in the Congee with Eggs and Spinach (page 25), Browned Butter Risotto (page 42), or Artichoke and Spinach Risotto (page 82). Use the remaining coconut milk in the Vegetable Korma (page 86).

SERVES 2

PREP & FINISHING:
5 MINUTES

PRESSURE COOK:
20 MINUTES HIGH

RELEASE:
NATURAL
10 MINUTES,
THEN QUICK

TOTAL TIME:
45 MINUTES

Per Serving
Calories: 438; Fat: 29 g;
Carbohydrates: 44 g;
Fiber: 4 g; Protein: 12 g;
Sodium: 98 mg

Lemon Mousse

I love all things lemon, especially lemon curd. But it's pretty intense on its own, so I often lighten it up with whipped cream to make an easy mousse. It goes especially well with gingersnaps on the side.

⅓ cup plus 2 teaspoons sugar
2 tablespoons unsalted butter, at room temperature
2 large egg yolks
Zest of 1 lemon

3 tablespoons freshly squeezed lemon juice (1 to 2 large lemons)
Pinch kosher salt
½ cup heavy (whipping) cream

MAKES 2 LARGE
OR 4 SMALL
SERVINGS

PREP & FINISHING:
15 MINUTES

PRESSURE COOK:
10 MINUTES HIGH

RELEASE:
NATURAL
10 MINUTES,
THEN QUICK

TOTAL TIME:
45 MINUTES,
PLUS 2 HOURS
TO CHILL

Per Serving
Calories: 554; Fat: 38 g;
Carbohydrates: 53 g;
Fiber: 0 g; Protein: 4 g;
Sodium: 195 mg

1. In a heat-proof bowl that will fit in the inner pot, beat the sugar and butter with a hand mixer until the sugar has mostly dissolved and the mixture is light colored and fluffy. Add the egg yolks and beat until combined. Add the lemon zest, lemon juice, and salt, and beat to combine. The mixture will appear grainy. Cover the bowl with aluminum foil.

2. Add 1 cup of water to the inner pot. Place a trivet with handles in the pot and then place the bowl on top. Lock the lid into place. Select Pressure Cook or Manual, and adjust the pressure to High and the time to 10 minutes. After cooking, let the pressure release naturally for 10 minutes, then quick release any remaining pressure. Unlock the lid. Carefully remove the bowl, and remove and discard the foil. The mixture will appear clumpy and curdled.

3. Whisk the curd mixture until smooth. Place a fine-mesh strainer over a medium bowl and pour the curd through it, pressing down with a flexible spatula to pass the curd through, leaving the zest and any curdled egg bits behind (discard those). Cover with plastic wrap, pushing the wrap down on top of the curd to keep a skin from forming. Refrigerate until cooled, about 2 hours.

4. When the curd is cooled, whip the cream until medium-firm peaks form. Add about a third of the whipped cream to the curd and fold it in gently. Repeat with another third of whipped cream, then finish with the last third. Spoon the mousse into dessert dishes and serve immediately, or refrigerate, covered, up to overnight.

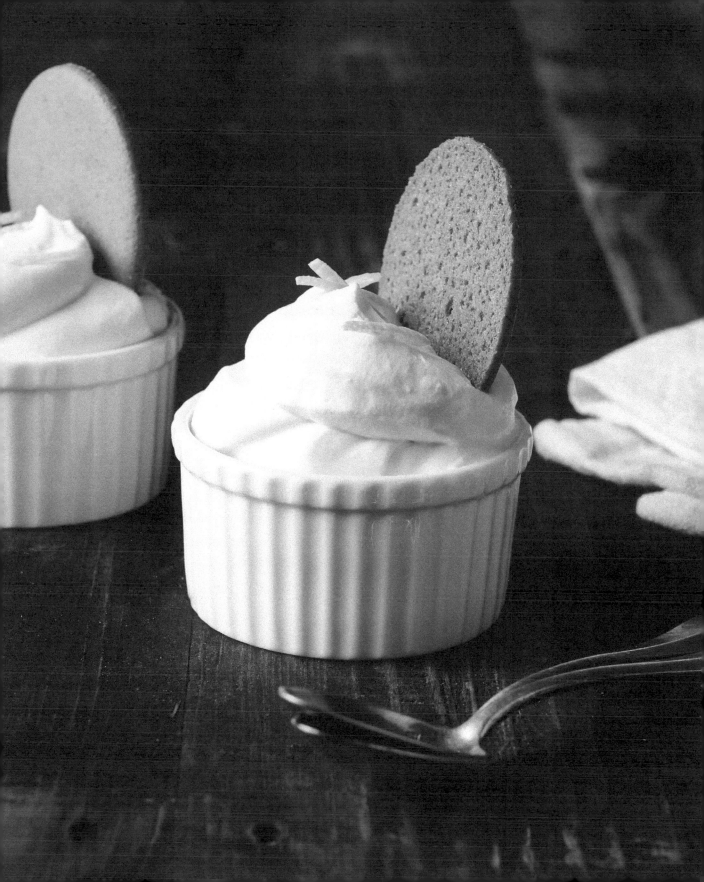

Mini Chocolate Marble Cheesecakes

There's nothing quite like chocolate cheesecake to end a romantic meal. Oh, let's be honest: There's nothing quite like chocolate cheesecake, period. And making these mini versions is fast and easy—no overnight chilling required. The swirl of vanilla batter on top of chocolate reverses the usual marble effect and is particularly beautiful. I like to use Guittard brand 60 percent chocolate chips, but any dark chocolate chips will work.

MAKES 4 SMALL
CHEESECAKES

PREP & FINISHING:
15 MINUTES

PRESSURE COOK:
6 MINUTES HIGH

RELEASE:
NATURAL
8 MINUTES,
THEN QUICK

TOTAL TIME:
40 MINUTES,
PLUS 20 MINUTES
TO COOL AND
4 HOURS TO CHILL

Per Serving
Calories: 432; Fat: 30 g;
Carbohydrates: 38 g;
Fiber: 1 g; Protein: 7 g;
Sodium: 267 mg

For the crust

½ cup chocolate wafer cookie crumbs (about 12 cookies, depending on size)

2 tablespoons unsalted butter, melted

For the filling

6 ounces cream cheese, at room temperature

1 tablespoon sour cream

½ teaspoon pure vanilla extract

¼ cup sugar

1 large egg

3 ounces dark chocolate chips, melted

To make the crust

Mix the cookie crumbs with the butter. Scoop out about 2 tablespoons of the crumb mixture into each of four (1-cup) ramekins or custard cups and press it down to make a layer a scant ¼ inch thick. You may not need all the crumbs, but you can reserve them and sprinkle over the top of the cheesecakes as garnish.

To make the filling

1. In a small bowl, beat the cream cheese, sour cream, and vanilla with a hand mixer until smooth. Add the sugar gradually, continuing to beat until the mixture is smooth again.

2. Beat in the egg until fully incorporated. Spoon out 2 tablespoons of the batter into a small bowl, then mix in the melted chocolate into the larger amount of batter.

3. Divide the chocolate cheesecake batter among the ramekins. Spoon the reserved vanilla batter over the chocolate mixture and swirl a skewer or small knife through it to create a marble pattern.

To make the cheesecakes

1. Add 1 cup of water to the inner pot. Place a trivet in the pot and then place the ramekins on top. If they won't all fit in one layer, it's fine to stack them. Drape a piece of foil over the ramekins to keep condensation off the top of the cheesecakes. Lock the lid in place.

2. Select Pressure Cook or Manual, and adjust the pressure to High and the time to 6 minutes. After cooking, let the pressure release naturally for 8 minutes, then quick release any remaining pressure.

3. Unlock the lid. Use tongs to remove the ramekins. Let cool for 20 minutes or so, then refrigerate to chill thoroughly, 3 to 4 hours.

Easier Together: One person can make and assemble the crusts while the other person works on the filling.

Make It Gluten-Free: Use gluten-free cookies for the crumbs.

Ricotta Cheesecakes
with Balsamic Strawberries

Strawberries, balsamic, and black pepper might seem like an odd combination, but trust me—they're amazing together. They complement these creamy cheesecakes perfectly. If you can't find good balsamic, or it's not strawberry season, the Mixed Berry Compote (page 167) is also a fine topping.

MAKES 4 SMALL
CHEESECAKES

PREP & FINISHING:
15 MINUTES

PRESSURE COOK:
6 MINUTES HIGH

RELEASE:
NATURAL
8 MINUTES,
THEN QUICK

TOTAL TIME:
30 MINUTES,
PLUS 20 MINUTES
TO COOL AND
4 HOURS TO CHILL

Per Serving
Calories: 300; Fat: 20 g;
Carbohydrates: 25 g;
Fiber: 1 g; Protein: 7 g;
Sodium: 135 mg

For the cheesecakes

4 ounces cream cheese

¼ cup heavy (whipping) cream

⅓ cup whole-milk ricotta cheese,
 at room temperature

⅓ cup sugar

1 teaspoon vanilla

1 large egg

1 egg yolk

Nonstick cooking spray

For the topping

⅔ cup sliced strawberries

2 teaspoons aged balsamic
 vinegar (I like Villa
 Manodori brand)

1 teaspoon sugar

Pinch freshly ground
 black pepper

To make the cheesecakes

1. In a small bowl, beat the cream cheese and cream with a hand mixer until smooth. Add the ricotta, sugar, and vanilla, and beat until the mixture is smooth again. Beat in the egg and egg yolk until fully incorporated.

2. With the cooking spray, generously spray four (6-ounce) ramekins. Divide the cheesecake batter among the ramekins.

3. Add 1 cup of water to the inner pot. Place a trivet in the pot and then place the ramekins on top. If they won't all fit in one layer, it's fine to layer them. Cover each with aluminum foil, but don't crimp it down.

4. Lock the lid in place. Select Pressure Cook or Manual, and adjust the pressure to High and the time to 6 minutes. After cooking, let the pressure release naturally for 8 minutes, then quick release any remaining pressure.

5. Unlock the lid. Use tongs to remove the ramekins. Let cool for 20 minutes or so, then refrigerate to chill thoroughly, 3 to 4 hours.

6. While the cheesecakes chill, prepare the topping.

To make the topping

In a small bowl, stir together all the ingredients.

To serve

1. Run a knife around the inside of each ramekin. Unmold by placing a plate over each ramekin and turning it upside down so that the cheesecake pops out (or if you prefer, you can serve the cakes in the ramekins).

2. Top with the balsamic strawberries and serve.

Use It Up: Use the leftover ricotta cheese in the Savory Ham and Cheese Egg Cups (page 35) or the Mixed-Up Lasagna (page 133). Leftover strawberries can go in the Mixed Berry Compote (page 167).

Carrot Cake

For the longest time, I thought I didn't like carrot cake. Turns out, I just don't like all the nuts and dried fruits that some people seem compelled to cram in the batter. (I do, however, like crystalized ginger, so if you have some left over from the Ginger-Oatmeal Muffins on page 23, it makes a nice addition.) Also, when you eat carrot cake, you get to eat cream cheese frosting! My frosting recipe makes a generous amount, but it's virtually impossible to whip less than ¼ cup of cream, so we just have to make do with more.

MAKES 4
SMALL SLICES

PREP & FINISHING:
25 MINUTES

PRESSURE COOK:
15 MINUTES HIGH

RELEASE:
NATURAL
9 MINUTES,
THEN QUICK

TOTAL TIME:
1 HOUR, PLUS
30 MINUTES
TO COOL

Per Serving
Calories: 562; Fat: 36 g;
Carbohydrates: 57 g;
Fiber: 1 g; Protein: 7 g;
Sodium: 472 mg

For the carrot cake

½ cup all-purpose flour, plus more for dusting

½ teaspoon baking soda

⅛ teaspoon kosher salt

½ teaspoon ground cinnamon

¼ teaspoon ground nutmeg

¼ teaspoon ground ginger or 1 tablespoon finely chopped crystalized ginger

½ cup sugar

¼ cup canola oil

2 tablespoons freshly squeezed orange juice

1 large egg

¾ cup finely grated carrots

Nonstick cooking spray

For the frosting

¼ cup heavy (whipping) cream

6 ounces cream cheese, at room temperature

½ cup powdered sugar

⅛ teaspoon grated orange zest (optional)

½ teaspoon vanilla

To make the carrot cake

1. In a medium bowl, whisk together the flour, baking soda, salt, cinnamon, nutmeg, and ginger. In a large bowl, whisk together the sugar, canola oil, and orange juice. Then, in the large bowl, add the egg and mix thoroughly. Add the flour mixture to the wet ingredients and stir until blended. Stir in the carrots.

2. Grease the bottom of a 6-inch cake pan with cooking spray and insert a round of parchment paper in the bottom. Spray the paper and sides of the pan with cooking spray and then dust with a thin layer of flour. Pour the batter into the pan and cover with aluminum foil.

3. Add 1 cup of water to the inner pot. Place a trivet with handles in the pot and then place the pan on top. Lock the lid into place.

Select Pressure Cook or Manual, and adjust the pressure to High and the time to 15 minutes. After cooking, let the pressure release naturally for 9 minutes, then quick release any remaining pressure.

4. Unlock the lid. Remove the cake and trivet. Remove the foil. Let cool for 30 to 60 minutes, then remove the cake from the pan.

To make the frosting

1. In a small, deep bowl, add the cream. With a hand mixer, whip the cream to form medium-stiff peaks. Set aside.

2. In a large bowl, beat the cream cheese until smooth. Add the powdered sugar, orange zest (if using), and vanilla and beat with a hand mixer until smooth.

3. Scoop about a third of the whipped cream onto the top of the cream cheese mixture. Gently fold it in with a flexible spatula. When the cream is incorporated into the cream cheese mixture, repeat with a second third of the whipped cream. Once incorporated, finish with the remaining whipped cream.

To serve

Spread the frosting over the top and sides of the cake (you may not need it all) and serve.

Double It: If you'd like to make a layered cake (to use up all that frosting), double the batter, then bake half of the cakes at a time. Empty the hot water after the first cake is baked. Let the pot cool, then add a fresh cup of water before baking the second layer.

Make It Dairy-Free: The cake itself is dairy-free, so for a dairy-free dessert, you can leave off the frosting and make an orange glaze instead. Sift about ½ a cup powdered sugar into 1 tablespoon freshly squeezed orange juice, adjusting the amounts until the consistency is to your liking. Drizzle over the cooled cake. Or, if you prefer, you can top it with Small-Batch Applesauce (page 166).

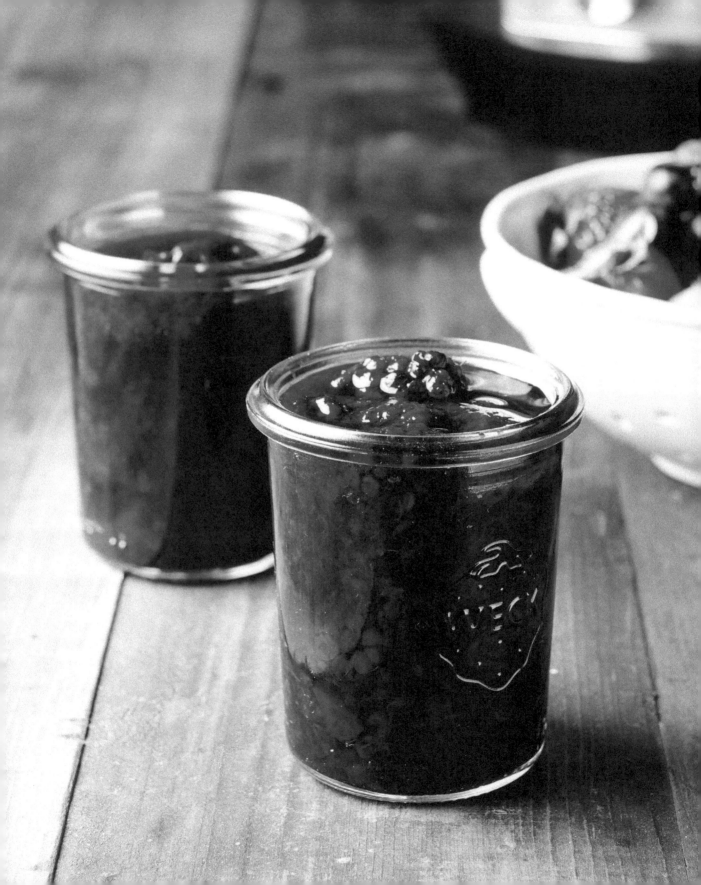

chapter 9
Kitchen Staples

Chicken Stock . . . 158

Mushroom Stock . . . 159

Marinara Sauce . . . 160

Basic Beans . . . 162

Basic White or Brown Rice . . . 163

Small-Batch Yogurt . . . 164

Small-Batch Applesauce . . . 166

Mixed Berry Compote . . . 167

Mixed Berry Compote, page 167

Chicken Stock

While pressure-cooked chicken stock does take time, it's still much faster than when cooked on the stove top, and it requires no supervision. In two hours, you'll have deeply flavored stock with a beautiful texture. Many recipes for chicken stock or broth call for the addition of vegetables and herbs, but I prefer to make it without them, as they tend to become bitter with long cooking.

MAKES 1 QUART
[½ CUP = 1 SERVING]

PREP & FINISHING:
20 MINUTES

PRESSURE COOK:
90 MINUTES HIGH

RELEASE:
NATURAL
15 MINUTES,
THEN QUICK

TOTAL TIME:
2 HOURS

Per Serving
Calories: 10; Fat: 0 g;
Carbohydrates: 1 g;
Fiber: 0 g; Protein: 1 g;
Sodium: 25 mg

2 pounds meaty chicken bones (backs, wing tips, leg quarters)

¼ teaspoon kosher salt
3½ cups water

1. Place the chicken parts in the inner pot and sprinkle with the salt. Add the water; don't worry if it doesn't cover the bones.

2. Select Pressure Cook or Manual, and adjust the pressure to High and the time to 90 minutes. After cooking, let the pressure release naturally for 15 minutes, then quick release any remaining pressure. Unlock the lid.

3. Line a colander with cheesecloth and place it over a large bowl. Pour the chicken parts and stock into the colander to strain out the chicken and bones. Let the stock cool and then refrigerate for several hours or overnight so that the fat hardens on top of the stock. Peel off the fat. Refrigerated, the stock will last several days, or it can be frozen for up to a month.

Use In: Any recipes that call for chicken stock or broth, especially Chicken Noodle Soup (page 115).

Mushroom Stock

I first read about this method of making mushroom stock in the book Modernist Cuisine, *and thought it couldn't be as good as everyone said it was. Was I ever wrong! It still amazes me that nothing but mushrooms and browned shallots can produce this much flavor in a couple of hours.*

1 tablespoon extra-virgin olive oil

4 ounces shallots, thinly sliced (about 4 medium shallot bulbs)

1 pound cremini or white button mushrooms, sliced

⅛ teaspoon kosher salt

3½ cups water

1. Select Sauté and adjust to Medium heat. Add the olive oil to the inner pot and heat until it shimmers. Add the shallots and cook, stirring, until the shallots are quite brown, about 5 minutes. Add the mushrooms, salt, and water to the pot.

2. Lock the lid into place. Select Pressure Cook or Manual, and adjust the pressure to High and the time to 45 minutes. After cooking, let the pressure release naturally for 15 minutes, then quick release any remaining pressure.

3. Unlock the lid. Pour the contents through a fine-mesh strainer into a large bowl. Discard the mushrooms and shallots. Let the stock cool for 20 minutes or so, then refrigerate. Leftover stock will keep in the refrigerator for several days, or it can be frozen for up to a month.

Use In: Mushroom Stroganoff (page 83) or any recipe that calls for vegetable stock.

MAKES 1 QUART
[½ CUP = 1 SERVING]

PREP & FINISHING:
10 MINUTES

SAUTÉ:
5 MINUTES

PRESSURE COOK:
45 MINUTES HIGH

RELEASE:
NATURAL
15 MINUTES,
THEN QUICK

TOTAL TIME:
1 HOUR
30 MINUTES

Per Serving
Calories: 10; Fat: 0 g;
Carbohydrates: 2 g;
Fiber: 1 g; Protein: 1 g;
Sodium: 32 mg

Marinara Sauce

Making your own marinara sauce isn't difficult and the result is more delicious and much less expensive than commercial brands. Sun-dried tomatoes aren't traditional, but I think they give a deeper tomato flavor to the sauce.

3 tablespoons extra-virgin olive oil

½ small onion, minced (about ¼ cup)

2 garlic cloves, minced

1 tablespoon minced or puréed sun-dried tomatoes

1 (14-ounce) can crushed tomatoes

½ teaspoon dried oregano

Pinch red pepper flakes

½ teaspoon kosher salt

MAKES ABOUT 2 CUPS
[¼ CUP = 1 SERVING]

PREP & FINISHING:
5 MINUTES

SAUTÉ:
4 MINUTES

PRESSURE COOK:
12 MINUTES HIGH

RELEASE:
NATURAL
10 MINUTES,
THEN QUICK

TOTAL TIME:
40 MINUTES

Per Serving
Calories: 74; Fat: 6 g;
Carbohydrates: 5 g;
Fiber: 2 g; Protein: 1 g;
Sodium: 174 mg

1. Select Sauté and adjust to High heat. Add the olive oil to the pot and heat until it shimmers. Add the onion and garlic. Cook, stirring, for 2 to 3 minutes, or until the vegetables start to soften. Add the sun-dried tomatoes and cook for 1 minute, or until fragrant.

2. Pour in the crushed tomatoes and stir to combine, scraping the bottom of the pot to loosen any vegetables that might be stuck. Stir in the oregano, red pepper flakes, and salt.

3. Lock the lid in place. Select Pressure Cook or Manual, and adjust the pressure to High and the time to 12 minutes. After cooking, release the pressure naturally for 10 minutes, then quick release any remaining pressure. Unlock the lid.

4. Let the sauce cool for about 10 minutes, then taste and adjust the seasoning, adding more salt if necessary. Refrigerate for up to a week or freeze for 4 to 6 weeks.

Use In: Mixed-Up Lasagna (page 133), or serve over polenta instead of the Mushroom Sauce (page 78). Marinara makes a great sauce on pizza or pasta as well.

Use It Up: Use leftover sun-dried tomatoes in the Rotini with Creamy Basil and Sun-Dried Tomato Sauce (page 81).

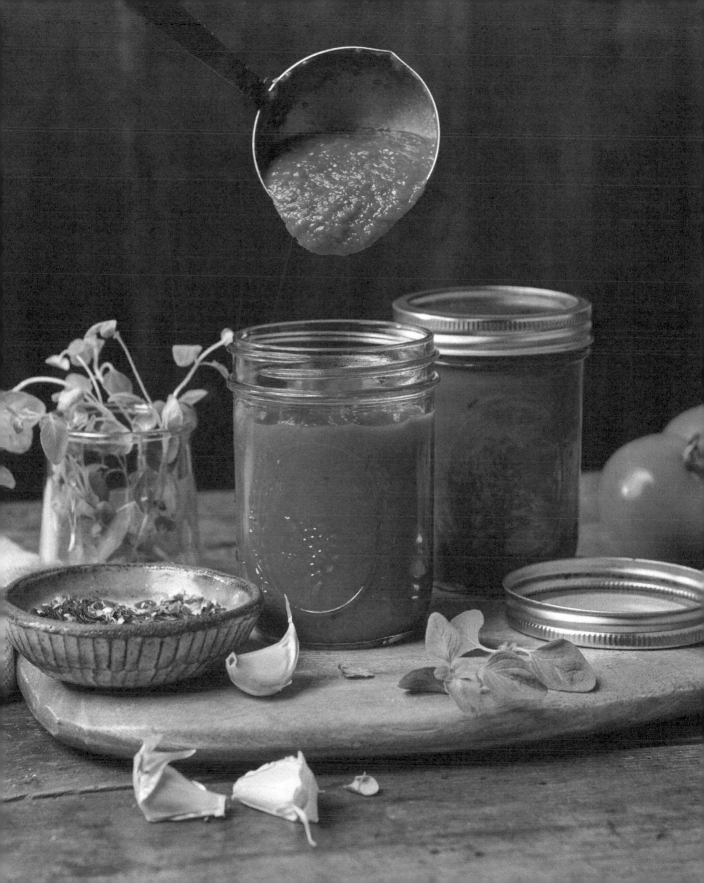

Basic Beans

While I've included several recipes for various kinds of beans, this one is great when you just want to cook plain beans to use in your own recipes. Different types of dried beans will yield slightly different volumes of cooked beans, but here are some ballpark amounts: 2 ounces of dried beans (about ⅓ cup) will yield a little less than 1 cup when cooked; 3 ounces (about ½ cup) will yield slightly more than 1 cup cooked beans. To make about the same amount of beans as in a 15-ounce can, start with 4 ounces, or about a ⅔ cup of beans. (See the tip to multiply the recipe.)

MAKES ABOUT 1 CUP
[¼ CUP = 1 SERVING]

PREP & FINISHING:
10 MINUTES

PRESSURE COOK:
8 MINUTES HIGH

RELEASE:
NATURAL
10 MINUTES,
THEN QUICK

TOTAL TIME:
35 MINUTES,
PLUS 8 HOURS
TO SOAK

Per Serving
Calories: 84; Fat: 0 g;
Carbohydrates: 15 g;
Fiber: 4 g; Protein: 5 g;
Sodium: 78 mg

2 or 3 ounces dried pinto, black, small red, navy, or cannellini beans (⅓ to ½ cup)

3 cups water, divided

2 teaspoons kosher salt, divided

1. Pour the beans into a small bowl. Add 2 cups of water and 1½ teaspoons of salt. Let soak at room temperature for 6 to 8 hours. Drain and rinse.

2. Pour the soaked beans into the inner pot. Add the remaining 1 cup of water and ½ teaspoon of salt. Lock the lid into place. Select Pressure Cook or Manual, and adjust the pressure to High and the time to 8 minutes. After cooking, let the pressure release naturally for 10 minutes, then quick release the remaining pressure.

3. Unlock the lid. Drain the beans, then cool and refrigerate if not using immediately.

Double It: You can cook up to 8 ounces of dried beans at a time. For 4 to 8 ounces of beans, use 1 quart water plus 1 tablespoon salt to soak. For cooking, use 1 cup of water and ½ teaspoon of salt per 2 or 3 ounces of dried beans.

Use In: Use cooked pinto beans in Easy Chili (page 123), cooked black beans in Southwestern Black Bean Salad (page 60), or cooked white beans in the Italian Tuna and Bean Salad (page 102).

Basic White or Brown Rice

Yes, the Instant Pot® has a rice setting, and yes, it works well in some cases. But it's designed to work with white rice only, and no less than 1 cup of rice. So when you're cooking for two, or cooking brown rice—or both—that setting is often not your best bet. This method works with as little as ½ cup of either type of rice, which cooks into enough for two generous servings—between 1⅔ and 1¾ cups.

½ cup long-grain white or brown rice

½ cup water

¼ teaspoon kosher salt

1. Pour the rice into a strainer, rinse it with cold water, and then drain.

2. Pour the rinsed rice into the inner pot. Add the water and salt. Stir to dissolve the salt.

3. Lock the lid into place. Select Pressure Cook or Manual, and adjust the pressure to High and the time to 4 minutes for white rice or 22 minutes for brown rice. After cooking, let the pressure release naturally for 10 minutes, then quick release any remaining pressure.

4. Unlock the lid. Fluff the rice with a fork and taste; if it's not quite done, just replace the lid (not locked) and let it steam for a few more minutes.

Double It: Double all the ingredients, but keep the cooking time the same.

Use In: Sweet and Sour Chicken (page 114), Spicy Braised Tofu and Carrots (page 80), Vegetable Korma (page 86), Char Siu (page 134), and Korean Short Ribs (page 122).

SERVES 2

PREP & FINISHING:
3 MINUTES

PRESSURE COOK:
WHITE:
4 MINUTES HIGH

BROWN:
22 MINUTES HIGH

RELEASE:
NATURAL
10 MINUTES,
THEN QUICK

TOTAL TIME:
25 MINUTES FOR
WHITE RICE;
40 MINUTES FOR
BROWN RICE

Per Serving
Calories: 50; Fat: 0 g;
Carbohydrates: 9 g;
Fiber: 0 g; Protein: 1 g;
Sodium: 75 mg

Small-Batch Yogurt

There are several different ways to make yogurt in an Instant Pot®, but I find this to be the most reliable, least expensive, and easiest. Starting with just a quart of milk means it heats up to the right temperature without fail the first time through on the yogurt setting. If you start it in the evening, it can ferment overnight. In the morning, cover the inner pot, place it in the refrigerator, and you'll have perfect yogurt when you come home from work.

MAKES ABOUT 4 CUPS
[½ CUP = 1 SERVING]

PREP:
5 MINUTES

YOGURT SETTING:
ABOUT 25 MINUTES
PLUS 8 TO 10 HOURS

TOTAL TIME:
9 TO 11 HOURS,
PLUS 4 HOURS
TO COOL

Per Serving
Calories: 74; Fat: 4 g;
Carbohydrates: 6 g;
Fiber: 0 g; Protein: 4 g;
Sodium: 50 mg

1 quart whole milk

1 tablespoon plain whole-milk yogurt with live cultures, at room temperature

1. Add the milk to the inner pot. Select Yogurt and adjust so that BOIL shows in the display. Lock the lid into place. When the beeper sounds, unlock the lid. Use a thermometer to take the temperature of the milk in the center of the pot. It should read between 179°F and 182°F.

2. Fill a large bowl or the sink with ice water and place the inner pot in it to cool. Stir the milk occasionally, without scraping the bottom of the pot, for about 3 minutes, then take the temperature in the center of the milk again. It should read between 110°F and 115°F. Remove the pot from the ice bath and dry off the outside of the pot.

3. In a small bowl, stir together the yogurt and about ½ cup of the warm milk. Add the yogurt mixture to the pot and stir thoroughly but gently. Again, don't scrape the bottom of the pot (if there is any coagulated milk on the bottom, stirring it in can make your finished yogurt less smooth).

4. Lock the lid into place (or use a glass lid) and select Yogurt. The display should read 8:00, which indicates 8 hours of incubation time. If you prefer a longer incubation, press the [+] button to increase the time by increments of 30 minutes. When the yogurt cycle is complete, remove the inner pot and cover it with a glass or silicone lid, or place a plate on top. Refrigerate until cool, about 4 hours, before using or stirring.

5. For Greek yogurt: Line a colander or large sieve with cheesecloth. Place the colander over a large bowl. Spoon the yogurt into the colander and let drain for 15 to 30 minutes, depending on how thick you want your yogurt.

Use In: Any recipes calling for yogurt or Greek yogurt, such as Shawarma-Style Chicken and Rice (page 106), Ginger-Oatmeal Muffins (page 23), and Beet Salad with Creamy Dill Dressing (page 44). Mix the yogurt with Small-Batch Applesauce (page 166) or Mixed Berry Compote (page 167) for a quick breakfast.

Small-Batch Applesauce

Making your own applesauce is easy, and despite what many recipes call for, you don't have to make a huge batch. I like the subtle flavors that whole spices give the sauce, but you can skip them and add ground spices after cooking if you like, or leave them out if you prefer your applesauce plain.

1½ pounds apples, such as McIntosh, Gala, or Jonathan

3 tablespoons unsweetened apple juice or apple cider

1 tablespoon brown sugar

1 tablespoon freshly squeezed lemon juice

Pinch kosher salt

1 small cinnamon stick (optional)

2 or 3 whole cloves or whole cardamom pods (optional)

MAKES ABOUT 2 CUPS
[¼ CUP = 1 SERVING]

PREP & FINISHING:
15 MINUTES

PRESSURE COOK:
4 MINUTES HIGH

RELEASE:
NATURAL
15 MINUTES,
THEN QUICK

TOTAL TIME:
45 MINUTES

Per Serving
Calories: 106; Fat: 0 g;
Carbohydrates: 28 g;
Fiber: 5 g; Protein: 1 g;
Sodium: 22 mg

1. Peel, halve, and core the apples. Cut each apple half into 4 wedges and cut each wedge in half crosswise.

2. Place the apples in the inner pot. Add the apple juice, brown sugar, lemon juice, salt, and cinnamon stick and cloves (if using). Stir to combine.

3. Lock the lid in place. Select Pressure Cook or Manual, and adjust the pressure to High and the time to 4 minutes. After cooking, release the pressure naturally for 15 minutes, then quick release any remaining pressure.

4. Unlock the lid. Remove and discard the cinnamon stick and cloves. Use a potato masher to break up the apples if you like chunky applesauce, or purée with an immersion blender if you prefer a smoother sauce. Taste and adjust the seasoning, adding more sugar if desired.

Use In: Stir into the Steel-Cut Oatmeal with Cranberries and Almonds (page 22) after cooking, or spoon over the Carrot Cake (page 154) instead of frosting it.

Mixed Berry Compote

This compote is a delicious, versatile fruit mixture you can use in breakfasts or desserts. Because different berries have different sweetness levels, I start with a fairly small amount of sugar before cooking and adjust as necessary afterward. The fruits start to release liquid almost immediately when you mix them with sugar, so no extra liquid is needed for the cooking process.

4 cups fresh berries, such as strawberries, raspberries, blueberries, or blackberries

¼ cup sugar, or more as needed

1 teaspoon freshly squeezed lemon juice

1 teaspoon orange juice concentrate (optional)

1. If you're using strawberries, remove the stems and cut the berries in halves or quarters, depending on size. Wash all the berries.

2. Add the berries and sugar to the inner pot. Stir to start dissolving the sugar. Add the lemon juice and orange juice concentrate (if using).

3. Lock the lid in place. Select Pressure Cook or Manual, and adjust the pressure to High and the time to 2 minutes. After cooking, let the pressure release naturally for 10 minutes, then quick release any remaining pressure.

4. Unlock the lid. Taste the berries (carefully—they're hot) and adjust the sugar if necessary. The berries will be soupy, but will thicken up slightly as they cool. If you prefer a thicker compote, you can strain off some of the juice (it's great mixed into sparkling water) or cook the fruit further to evaporate some of the liquid.

Double It: Double all ingredients, keeping the cooking time the same.

Use In: You can top the Ricotta Cheesecakes (page 152) with these berries instead of the balsamic strawberries, mix into the Steel-Cut Oatmeal with Cranberries and Almonds (page 22) after cooking, or stir the compote into Small-Batch Yogurt (page 164).

MAKES ABOUT 2 CUPS [¼ CUP = 1 SERVING]

PREP & FINISHING:
15 MINUTES

PRESSURE COOK:
2 MINUTES HIGH

RELEASE:
NATURAL
10 MINUTES,
THEN QUICK

TOTAL TIME:
35 MINUTES

Per Serving
Calories: 60; Fat: 0 g;
Carbohydrates: 15 g;
Fiber: 3 g; Protein: 1 g;
Sodium: 1 mg

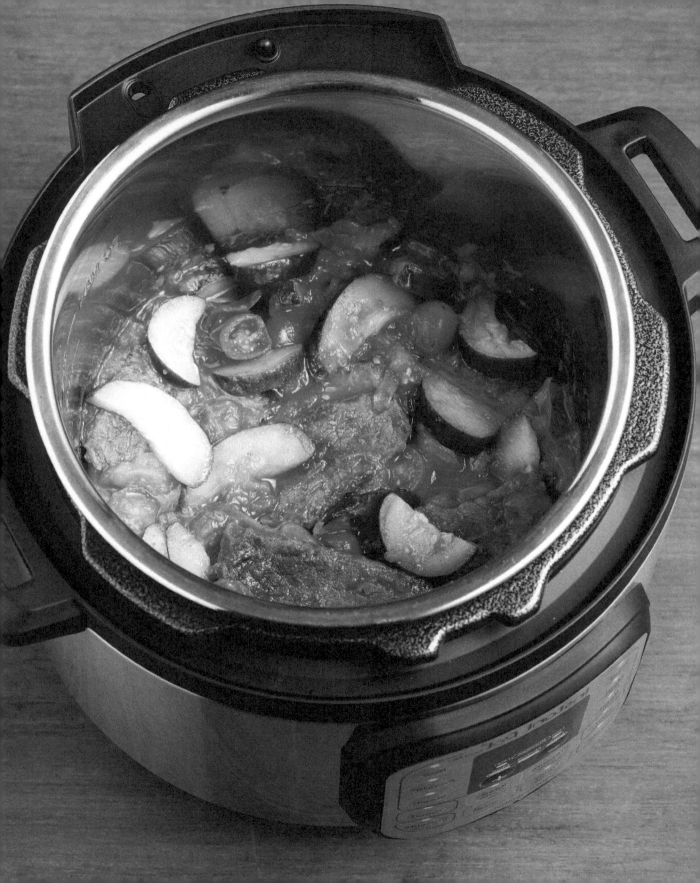

Instant Pot® Pressure Cooking Time Charts

The following charts provide approximate pressure cook times for a variety of foods. To begin, you may want to cook for a minute or two less than the times listed; you can always simmer foods at natural release to finish cooking. The cooking times for the ingredients when they are part of a recipe may differ because of additional ingredients or cooking liquids or a different release method than the one listed here.

For any foods labeled Natural release, allow at least 15 minutes natural pressure release before releasing remaining pressure.

Fish and Seafood

All times are for steamed fish and shellfish.

	Minutes Under Pressure	Pressure	Release
Clams	2	High	Quick
Halibut (1 inch thick)	3	High	Quick
Mussels	1	High	Quick
Salmon (1 inch thick)	5	Low	Quick
Shrimp, large (frozen)	1	Low	Quick
Tilapia or cod (frozen)	3	Low	Quick

Poultry

Except as noted, these times are for braised poultry; that is, partially submerged in liquid.

	Minutes Under Pressure	Pressure	Release
Chicken breast, bone-in	8 (steamed)	Low	Natural 5 minutes, then Quick
Chicken breast, boneless	5 (steamed)	Low	Natural 8 minutes, then Quick
Chicken thigh, bone-in	12 to 15	High	Natural 10 minutes, then Quick
Chicken thigh, boneless, whole	8	High	Natural 10 minutes, then Quick
Chicken thigh, 1- to 2-inch pieces	5 to 6	High	Quick
Chicken, whole (seared on all sides)	14 to 18	Low	Natural 8 minutes, then Quick
Duck quarters, bone-in	35	High	Quick
Turkey breast, tenderloin (12 ounces)	5 (steamed)	Low	Natural 8 minutes, then Quick
Turkey thigh, bone-in	30	High	Natural

Meat

Except as noted, these times are for braised meats; that is, meats that are seared before pressure cooking, and partially submerged in liquid.

	Minutes Under Pressure	Pressure	Release
Beef, shoulder (chuck) roast (2 pounds)	35 to 45	High	Natural
Beef, shoulder (chuck), 2-inch chunks	20	High	Natural 10 minutes, then Quick
Beef, bone-in short ribs	40	High	Natural
Beef, flat-iron steak, cut into ½-inch strips	6	Low	Quick
Beef, sirloin steak, cut into ½-inch strips	3	Low	Quick
Lamb, shanks	40	High	Natural
Lamb, shoulder, 2-inch chunks	35	High	Natural
Pork back ribs (steamed)	25	High	Quick
Pork spare ribs (steamed)	20	High	Quick
Pork shoulder roast (2 pounds)	25	High	Natural
Pork, shoulder, 2-inch chunks	20	High	Quick
Pork tenderloin	4	Low	Quick
Smoked pork sausage, ½-inch slices	5 to 10	High	Quick

Beans and Legumes

When cooking beans, if you have a pound or more, it's best to use low pressure and increase the cooking time by a minute or two (with larger amounts, there's more chance for foaming at high pressure). If you have less than a pound, high pressure is fine. A little oil in the cooking liquid will reduce foaming. Where two times are listed, the shorter time is for high pressure and the longer time for low pressure. (Beans and legumes should be soaked first for 8 to 24 hours in salted water unless otherwise noted.)

	Minutes Under Pressure	Pressure	Release
Black beans	8 or 9	Low or High	Natural
Black-eyed peas	5	High	Natural 8 minutes, then Quick
Cannellini beans	5 or 7	Low or High	Natural
Chickpeas (garbanzo beans)	4	High	Natural 3 minutes, then Quick
Kidney beans	5 or 7	Low or High	Natural
Lentils, brown (unsoaked)	20	High	Natural 10 minutes, then Quick
Lentils, red (unsoaked)	10	High	Natural 5 minutes, then Quick
Lima beans	4 or 5	Low or High	Natural 5 minutes, then Quick
Pinto beans	8 or 10	Low or High	Natural
Soybeans, dried	12 or 14	Low or High	Natural
Soybeans, fresh (edamame), unsoaked	1	High	Quick
Split peas (unsoaked)	5 to 8	Low or High	Natural

Grains

To prevent foaming, it's best to include a small amount of butter or oil with the cooking liquid for these grains or to rinse them thoroughly before cooking.

	Liquid per 1 cup of Grain	Minutes Under Pressure	Pressure	Release
Arborio (or other medium-grain) rice	1½ cups	6 to 20 (depending on use)	High	Quick
Barley, pearled	2½ cups	20	High	Natural 10 minutes, then Quick
Brown rice, long grain	1½ cups	13	High	Natural 10 minutes, then Quick
Brown rice, medium-grain	1½ cups	6 to 8	High	Natural
Buckwheat	1¾ cups	2 to 4	High	Natural
Farro, pearled	2 cups	6 to 8	High	Natural
Farro, whole-grain	3 cups	22 to 24	High	Natural
Oats, rolled	3 cups	3 to 4	High	Quick
Oats, steel-cut	4 cups	12	High	Natural
Quinoa	1½ cups	1	High	Natural 12 minutes, then Quick
Wheat berries	2 cups	30	High	Natural 10 minutes, then Quick
Long-grain white rice	1 cup	3	High	Natural
Wild rice	1¼ cups	22 to 24	High	Natural

Vegetables

The cooking method for the following vegetables is steaming; if the vegetables are cooked in liquid, the times may vary. Green vegetables will be tender-crisp; root vegetables will be soft.

	Prep	Minutes Under Pressure	Pressure	Release
Acorn squash	Halved	9	High	Quick
Artichokes, large	Whole	15	High	Quick
Beets	Quartered if large; halved if small	9	High	Natural
Broccoli	Cut into florets	1	Low	Quick
Brussels sprouts	Halved	2	High	Quick
Butternut squash	Peeled, cut into ½-into chunks	8	High	Quick
Cabbage	Sliced	5	High	Quick
Carrots	½- to 1-inch slices	2	High	Quick
Cauliflower	Whole	6	High	Quick
Cauliflower	Cut into florets	1	Low	Quick
Green beans	Cut in half or thirds	1	Low	Quick
Potatoes, large russet	Quartered; for mashing	8	High	Natural 8 minutes, then Quick
Potatoes, red	Whole if less than 1½ inch across, halved if larger	4	High	Quick
Spaghetti squash	Halved lengthwise	7	High	Quick
Sweet potatoes	Halved lengthwise	8	High	Natural

Measurement Conversions

Oven Temperatures

Fahrenheit (F)	Celsius (C) (approx.)
250°F	120°C
300°F	150°C
325°F	165°C
350°F	180°C
375°F	190°C
400°F	200°C
425°F	220°C
450°F	230°C

Weight Equivalents

Standard	Metric (approx.)
½ ounce	15 g
1 ounce	30 g
2 ounces	60 g
4 ounces	115 g
8 ounces	225 g
12 ounces	340 g
16 ounces or 1 pound	455 g

Volume Equivalents (Liquid)

Standard	US Standard (oz.)	Metric (approx.)
2 tablespoons	1 fl. oz.	30 mL
¼ cup	2 fl. oz.	60 mL
½ cup	4 fl. oz.	120 mL
1 cup	8 fl. oz.	240 mL
1½ cups	12 fl. oz.	355 mL
2 cups or 1 pint	16 fl. oz.	475 mL
4 cups or 1 quart	32 fl. oz.	1 L
1 gallon	128 fl. oz.	4 L

Volume Equivalents (Dry)

Standard	Metric (approx.)
⅛ teaspoon	0.5 mL
¼ teaspoon	1 mL
½ teaspoon	2 mL
¾ teaspoon	4 mL
1 teaspoon	5 mL
1 tablespoon	15 mL
¼ cup	59 mL
⅓ cup	79 mL
½ cup	118 mL
⅔ cup	156 mL
¾ cup	177 mL
1 cup	235 mL
2 cups or 1 pint	475 mL
3 cups	700 mL
4 cups or 1 quart	1 L

Recipe Index

A

Apple-Cinnamon French Toast Cups, 24
Artichoke and Spinach Risotto, 82
Asparagus with Balsamic and Pine Nuts, 49

B

Barbecue Chicken Sandwiches with Slaw, 116–117
Basic Beans, 162
Basic White or Brown Rice, 163
Beef Stew, 124–125
Beet Salad with Creamy Dill Dressing, 44
Broccoli Rabe with Lemon-Anchovy Vinaigrette, 52
Brown Rice and Broccoli Cheese Casserole, 61
Browned Butter Risotto, 42
Butter-Braised Cabbage and Carrots, 53

C

Carrot Cake, 154–155
Char Siu, 134–135
Chicken Noodle Soup, 115
Chicken Paprikash, 112
Chicken Stock, 158
Chicken Thighs with Salami and Fennel, 110–111
Chorizo and Green Chile Breakfast Casserole, 32–33
Cilantro-Coconut Shrimp and Broccoli, 100
Citrus Custard, 145
Clam Chowder, 96–97
Coconut-Vanilla Rice Pudding, 147
Cod and Green Beans with Dill Mustard Sauce, 94–95
Congee with Eggs and Spinach, 25
Creamy Mushroom-Barley Soup, 70
Creamy Salsa Verde Chicken, 105
Crispy Salt and Vinegar Potatoes, 38–39
Curried Cauliflower Soup, 76

E

Easy Chili, 123
Eggs "en Cocotte," 29–30

F

Farfalle with Salmon, Fennel, and Tomatoes, 92–93
French Onion Soup Dip Sandwiches, 126–127

G

German Potato Salad, 40–41
Ginger-Oatmeal Muffins, 23
Greek Salad with Bulgur Wheat, 62

H

Ham and Potato Soup, 140–141
Hard-Cooked Eggs Two Ways, 26–27
Herbed Wild Rice Pilaf with Almonds, 66

I

Italian Pork Sandwiches, 136–137
Italian Tuna and Bean Salad, 102–103

J

Jamaican Rice and Peas, 68–69

K

Kielbasa and Vegetable Stew, 131
Korean Short Ribs, 122

L

Lemon Mousse, 148
Lentils with Red Peppers and Feta, 67

M

Maple Nutmeg Custard, 144
Marinara Sauce, 160
Minestrone, 74–75
Mini Chocolate Marble Cheesecakes, 150–151
Mixed Berry Compote, 167
Mixed-Up Lasagna, 133

Mushroom Stock, 159
Mushroom Stroganoff, 83

N

North African Chickpea Stew, 57

P

Penne with Italian Sausage and Broccoli Rabe, 132
Perfect Chicken Breast, 104
Pimiento Cheese Corn Pudding, 43
Pinto Beans with Chorizo, 58–59
Polenta with Mushroom Sauce, 78–79
Pork Tacos with Pineapple Salsa, 138–139

Q

Quinoa with Marinated Artichokes and Peppers, 71

R

Rice Pilaf with Bacon and Water Chestnuts, 64–65
Ricotta Cheesecakes with Balsamic Strawberries, 152–153
Roasted Sweet Potatoes and Beets with Rosemary, 46
Rotini with Creamy Basil and Sun-Dried Tomato Sauce, 81

S

Savory Ham and Cheese Egg Cups, 35
Scalloped Potatoes with Smoked Salmon, 90–91
Shawarma-Style Chicken and Rice, 106–107
Shrimp and Grits, 98–99
Small-Batch Applesauce, 166
Small-Batch Yogurt, 164–165
Smashed Red Potatoes with Bacon, 48
Southwestern Black Bean Salad, 60
Spaghetti Squash with Browned Butter and Parmesan, 77

Spanish Tortilla, 31
Spiced Peach Bread Pudding, 146
Spicy Braised Tofu and Carrots, 80
Spicy Chicken Lettuce
    Cups, 108–109
Spicy Sesame Noodles and
    Vegetables, 85
Steel-Cut Oatmeal with
    Cranberries and Almonds, 22
Sweet and Sour Chicken, 114

T

Tangy Carrot and Celery Salad, 45
Teriyaki Chicken and Rice, 113
Thai Red Curry Beef, 129–130
Tomato, Mozzarella, and Basil
    Quiche, 34
Turkey and Stuffing for
    Two, 118–119

V

Vegetable Korma, 86–87

W

Warm Thai-Style Green Bean and
    Tomato Salad, 50–51
White Bean Stew with Broccoli
    Rabe, 56

Index

A

Almonds
Herbed Wild Rice Pilaf with
Almonds, 66
Spicy Chicken Lettuce
Cups, 108–109
Steel-Cut Oatmeal with
Cranberries and
Almonds, 22
Vegetable Korma, 86–87

Anchovy paste
Broccoli Rabe with
Lemon-Anchovy
Vinaigrette, 52
French Onion Soup Dip
Sandwiches, 126–127

Apples
Apple-Cinnamon French Toast
Cups, 24
Small-Batch Applesauce, 166

Artichoke hearts
Artichoke and Spinach
Risotto, 82
Quinoa with Marinated
Artichokes and Peppers, 71

Asparagus
Asparagus with Balsamic and
Pine Nuts, 49

Avocados
Hard-Cooked Eggs Two
Ways, 26–27

B

Bacon
Clam Chowder, 96–97
German Potato Salad, 40–41
Rice Pilaf with Bacon and
Water Chestnuts, 64–65
Shrimp and Grits, 98–99
Smashed Red Potatoes with
Bacon, 48
Turkey and Stuffing for
Two, 118–119
Balsamic vinegar. *See* Vinegar,
balsamic

Barley
Creamy Mushroom-Barley
Soup, 70

Basil
Italian Tuna and Bean
Salad, 102–103
Rotini with Creamy Basil and
Sun-Dried Tomato Sauce, 81
Thai Red Curry Beef, 129–130
Tomato, Mozzarella, and Basil
Quiche, 34
Warm Thai-Style Green Bean
and Tomato Salad, 50–51
Beans. *See also* Chickpeas;
Green beans
Basic Beans, 162
Easy Chili, 123
Italian Tuna and Bean
Salad, 102–103
Jamaican Rice and Peas, 68–69
Minestrone, 74–75
Pinto Beans with
Chorizo, 58–59
portion guidelines, 10
Southwestern Black Bean
Salad, 60
White Bean Stew with Broccoli
Rabe, 56
Beef, 11
Beef Stew, 124–125
Easy Chili, 123
French Onion Soup Dip
Sandwiches, 126–127
Korean Short Ribs, 122
Thai Red Curry Beef, 129–130
Beets
Beet Salad with Creamy Dill
Dressing, 44
Roasted Sweet Potatoes and
Beets with Rosemary, 46
Bell peppers. *See* Peppers, bell
Berries. *See also* Cranberries, dried
Mixed Berry Compote, 167
Ricotta Cheesecakes
with Balsamic
Strawberries, 152–153
Bread
Apple-Cinnamon French Toast
Cups, 24
Chorizo and Green Chile
Breakfast Casserole, 32–33

Hard-Cooked Eggs Two
Ways, 26–27
Spiced Peach Bread
Pudding, 146
Turkey and Stuffing for
Two, 118–119
Broccoli
Brown Rice and Broccoli
Cheese Casserole, 61
Cilantro-Coconut Shrimp and
Broccoli, 100
Broccoli rabe
Broccoli Rabe with
Lemon-Anchovy
Vinaigrette, 52
Italian Pork Sandwiches,
136–137
Penne with Italian Sausage and
Broccoli Rabe, 132
White Bean Stew with Broccoli
Rabe, 56
Bulgur wheat
Greek Salad with Bulgur
Wheat, 62
"Burn" message, 14

C

Cabbage
Barbecue Chicken Sandwiches
with Slaw, 116–117
Butter-Braised Cabbage and
Carrots, 53
Kielbasa and Vegetable
Stew, 131
Carrots
Barbecue Chicken
Sandwiches with
Slaw, 116–117
Beef Stew, 124–125
Butter-Braised Cabbage and
Carrots, 53
Carrot Cake, 154–155
Chicken Noodle Soup, 115
Creamy Mushroom-Barley
Soup, 70
Ham and Potato Soup, 140–141
Kielbasa and Vegetable
Stew, 131

Minestrone, 74–75
  Spicy Braised Tofu and
    Carrots, 80
  Spicy Sesame Noodles and
    Vegetables, 85
  Tangy Carrot and Celery
    Salad, 45
  Vegetable Korma, 86–87
  White Bean Stew with Broccoli
    Rabe, 56
Cashews
  Vegetable Korma, 86–87
  Warm Thai-Style Green Bean
    and Tomato Salad, 50–51
Cauliflower
  Curried Cauliflower Soup, 76
  Vegetable Korma, 86–87
Celery
  Chicken Noodle Soup, 115
  Clam Chowder, 96–97
  Creamy Mushroom-Barley
    Soup, 70
  German Potato Salad, 40–41
  Tangy Carrot and Celery
    Salad, 45
  Turkey and Stuffing for
    Two, 118–119
Cheddar cheese
  Brown Rice and Broccoli
    Cheese Casserole, 61
  Eggs "en Cocotte," 29–30
  Ham and Potato Soup, 140–141
  Pimiento Cheese Corn
    Pudding, 43
  Smashed Red Potatoes with
    Bacon, 48
Cheese. *See specific*
Chicken, 11
  Barbecue Chicken Sandwiches
    with Slaw, 116–117
  Chicken Noodle Soup, 115
  Chicken Paprikash, 112
  Chicken Stock, 158
  Chicken Thighs with Salami
    and Fennel, 110–111
  Creamy Salsa Verde
    Chicken, 105
  Perfect Chicken Breast, 104
  Shawarma-Style Chicken and
    Rice, 106–107

Spicy Chicken Lettuce
    Cups, 108–109
  Sweet and Sour Chicken, 114
  Teriyaki Chicken and Rice, 113
Chickpeas
  North African Chickpea
    Stew, 57
Chiles
  Barbecue Chicken
    Sandwiches with
    Slaw, 116–117
  Chorizo and Green Chile
    Breakfast Casserole, 32–33
  Jamaican Rice and Peas, 68–69
  Warm Thai-Style Green Bean
    and Tomato Salad, 50–51
Chives
  Curried Cauliflower Soup, 76
  Eggs "en Cocotte," 29–30
Chocolate
  Mini Chocolate Marble
    Cheesecakes, 150–151
Cilantro
  Cilantro-Coconut Shrimp and
    Broccoli, 100
  Pinto Beans with
    Chorizo, 58–59
  Pork Tacos with Pineapple
    Salsa, 138–139
  Southwestern Black Bean
    Salad, 60
  Spicy Chicken Lettuce
    Cups, 108–109
  Thai Red Curry Beef, 129–130
  Vegetable Korma, 86–87
  Warm Thai-Style Green Bean
    and Tomato Salad, 50–51
Clams
  Clam Chowder, 96–97
Coconut milk
  Cilantro-Coconut Shrimp and
    Broccoli, 100
  Coconut-Vanilla Rice
    Pudding, 147
  Jamaican Rice and Peas, 68–69
  Thai Red Curry Beef, 129–130
  Vegetable Korma, 86–87
Cod
  Cod and Green Beans with Dill
    Mustard Sauce, 94–95

Corn
  Pimiento Cheese Corn
    Pudding, 43
  Southwestern Black Bean
    Salad, 60
Cranberries, dried
  Steel-Cut Oatmeal with
    Cranberries and
    Almonds, 22
Cream cheese
  Carrot Cake, 154–155
  Mini Chocolate Marble
    Cheesecakes, 150–151
  Ricotta Cheesecakes
    with Balsamic
    Strawberries, 152–153

D

Dill
  Beet Salad with Creamy Dill
    Dressing, 44
  Cod and Green Beans with Dill
    Mustard Sauce, 94–95
  Scalloped Potatoes with
    Smoked Salmon, 90–91

E

Eggs
  Chorizo and Green Chile
    Breakfast Casserole, 32–33
  Citrus Custard, 145
  Congee with Eggs and
    Spinach, 25
  Eggs "en Cocotte," 29–30
  Hard-Cooked Eggs Two
    Ways, 26–27
  Lemon Mousse, 148
  Maple Nutmeg Custard, 144
  Mini Chocolate Marble
    Cheesecakes, 150–151
  Ricotta Cheesecakes
    with Balsamic
    Strawberries, 152–153
  Savory Ham and Cheese Egg
    Cups, 35
  Scalloped Potatoes with
    Smoked Salmon, 90–91
  Spanish Tortilla, 31
  Tomato, Mozzarella, and Basil
    Quiche, 34

F

Fennel
    Chicken Thighs with Salami
        and Fennel, 110–111
    Farfalle with Salmon, Fennel,
        and Tomatoes, 92–93
Feta cheese
    Greek Salad with Bulgur
        Wheat, 62
    Lentils with Red Peppers and
        Feta, 67
Fish
    Cod and Green Beans with Dill
        Mustard Sauce, 94–95
    Farfalle with Salmon, Fennel,
        and Tomatoes, 92–93
    Italian Tuna and Bean
        Salad, 102–103
    Scalloped Potatoes with
        Smoked Salmon, 90–91
Frozen foods, 12

G

Ginger
    Carrot Cake, 154–155
    Congee with Eggs and
        Spinach, 25
    Ginger-Oatmeal Muffins, 23
    Jamaican Rice and Peas,
        68–69
    Korean Short Ribs, 122
    Spicy Chicken Lettuce
        Cups, 108–109
    Sweet and Sour Chicken, 114
    Teriyaki Chicken and Rice, 113
Grains. *See also specific*
    portion guidelines, 10
Green beans
    Cod and Green Beans with Dill
        Mustard Sauce, 94–95
    Italian Tuna and Bean
        Salad, 102–103
    Warm Thai-Style Green Bean
        and Tomato Salad, 50–51
Gruyère cheese
    French Onion Soup Dip
        Sandwiches, 126–127
    Savory Ham and Cheese Egg
        Cups, 35

H

Ham
    Ham and Potato Soup, 140–141
    Savory Ham and Cheese Egg
        Cups, 35
    White Bean Stew with Broccoli
        Rabe, 56
High pressure, 4

I

Instant Pot®
    about, 2
    accessories, 9
    advantages of, 3
    Mini, 8
    models, 8
    prep and cooking steps, 4–5
    terminology, 3–4
    troubleshooting, 14–16

J

Jalapeños
    Cilantro-Coconut Shrimp and
        Broccoli, 100
    Easy Chili, 123
    Pork Tacos with Pineapple
        Salsa, 138–139
    Spicy Chicken Lettuce
        Cups, 108–109
    Vegetable Korma, 86–87

K

Keep warm setting, 4

L

Lemons
    Beet Salad with Creamy Dill
        Dressing, 44
    Broccoli Rabe with
        Lemon-Anchovy
        Vinaigrette, 52
    Citrus Custard, 145
    Greek Salad with Bulgur
        Wheat, 62
    Hard-Cooked Eggs Two
        Ways, 26–27
    Lemon Mousse, 148
    Lentils with Red Peppers and
        Feta, 67

    Mixed Berry Compote, 167
    North African Chickpea
        Stew, 57
    Shawarma-Style Chicken and
        Rice, 106–107
    Small-Batch Applesauce, 166
Lentils
    Lentils with Red Peppers and
        Feta, 67
Lettuce
    Spicy Chicken Lettuce
        Cups, 108–109
Limes
    Pork Tacos with Pineapple
        Salsa, 138–139
    Southwestern Black Bean
        Salad, 60
    Thai Red Curry Beef, 129–130
    Warm Thai-Style Green Bean
        and Tomato Salad, 50–51
Liquids, 15
Low pressure, 4

M

Milk
    Apple-Cinnamon French Toast
        Cups, 24
    Chorizo and Green Chile
        Breakfast Casserole, 32–33
    Ham and Potato Soup, 140–141
    Polenta with Mushroom
        Sauce, 78–79
    Scalloped Potatoes with
        Smoked Salmon, 90–91
    Shrimp and Grits, 98–99
    Small-Batch Yogurt, 164–165
    Spanish Tortilla, 31
    Spiced Peach Bread Pudding, 146
    Steel-Cut Oatmeal with
        Cranberries and
        Almonds, 22
    Tomato, Mozzarella, and Basil
        Quiche, 34
Mint
    Greek Salad with Bulgur
        Wheat, 62
Monterey Jack cheese
    Chorizo and Green Chile
        Breakfast Casserole, 32–33

Creamy Salsa Verde
Chicken, 105
Pinto Beans with
Chorizo, 58–59
Mozzarella cheese
Mixed-Up Lasagna, 133
Tomato, Mozzarella, and Basil
Quiche, 34
Mushrooms
Creamy Mushroom-Barley
Soup, 70
Eggs "en Cocotte," 29–30
Mushroom Stock, 159
Mushroom Stroganoff, 83
Polenta with Mushroom
Sauce, 78–79
Shrimp and Grits, 98–99

N
Natural release, 4
Noodles. See also Pasta
Chicken Noodle Soup, 115
Chicken Paprikash, 112
Cilantro-Coconut Shrimp and
Broccoli, 100
Mushroom Stroganoff, 83
Spicy Sesame Noodles and
Vegetables, 85
Nuts. See specific

O
Oats
Ginger-Oatmeal Muffins, 23
Steel-Cut Oatmeal with
Cranberries and
Almonds, 22
Olives, Kalamata
Greek Salad with Bulgur
Wheat, 62
Oranges
Carrot Cake, 154–155
Citrus Custard, 145
Pork Tacos with Pineapple
Salsa, 138–139
Oregano
Herbed Wild Rice Pilaf with
Almonds, 66
Roasted Sweet Potatoes and
Beets with Rosemary, 46

P
Parmesan cheese
Artichoke and Spinach
Risotto, 82
Broccoli Rabe with
Lemon-Anchovy
Vinaigrette, 52
Browned Butter Risotto, 42
Minestrone, 74–75
Mixed-Up Lasagna, 133
Polenta with Mushroom
Sauce, 78–79
Rotini with Creamy Basil and
Sun-Dried Tomato Sauce, 81
Spaghetti Squash with Browned
Butter and Parmesan, 77
White Bean Stew with Broccoli
Rabe, 56
Parsley
Butter-Braised Cabbage and
Carrots, 53
Chicken Noodle Soup, 115
German Potato Salad, 40–41
Greek Salad with Bulgur
Wheat, 62
Herbed Wild Rice Pilaf with
Almonds, 66
Italian Pork Sandwiches,
136–137
Kielbasa and Vegetable
Stew, 131
Lentils with Red Peppers and
Feta, 67
Mixed-Up Lasagna, 133
Mushroom Stroganoff, 83
Quinoa with Marinated
Artichokes and Peppers, 71
Shawarma-Style Chicken and
Rice, 106–107
Spaghetti Squash with
Browned Butter and
Parmesan, 77
White Bean Stew with Broccoli
Rabe, 56
Pasta
Farfalle with Salmon, Fennel,
and Tomatoes, 92–93
Minestrone, 74–75

Mixed-Up Lasagna, 133
Penne with Italian Sausage and
Broccoli Rabe, 132
portion guidelines, 10
Rotini with Creamy Basil and
Sun-Dried Tomato Sauce, 81
Peaches
Spiced Peach Bread
Pudding, 146
Peanuts
Spicy Chicken Lettuce
Cups, 108–109
Spicy Sesame Noodles and
Vegetables, 85
Pears
Korean Short Ribs, 122
Peas
Vegetable Korma, 86–87
Peas, snow
Rice Pilaf with Bacon and
Water Chestnuts, 64–65
Spicy Sesame Noodles and
Vegetables, 85
Peppers, bell
Chicken Paprikash, 112
Pork Tacos with Pineapple
Salsa, 138–139
Southwestern Black Bean
Salad, 60
Spicy Chicken Lettuce
Cups, 108–109
Spicy Sesame Noodles and
Vegetables, 85
Sweet and Sour Chicken, 114
Thai Red Curry Beef, 129–130
Peppers, roasted red
Lentils with Red Peppers and
Feta, 67
Pimiento Cheese Corn
Pudding, 43
Quinoa with Marinated
Artichokes and Peppers, 71
Pine nuts
Asparagus with Balsamic and
Pine Nuts, 49
Pineapple
Pork Tacos with Pineapple
Salsa, 138–139
Sweet and Sour Chicken, 114

Polenta
  Polenta with Mushroom
    Sauce, 78–79
  Shrimp and Grits, 98–99
Pork, 11. *See also* Bacon;
    Ham; Sausage
  Char Siu, 134–135
  Italian Pork Sandwiches, 136–137
  Pork Tacos with Pineapple
    Salsa, 138–139
Potatoes. *See also* Sweet potatoes
  Beef Stew, 124–125
  Clam Chowder, 96–97
  Crispy Salt and Vinegar
    Potatoes, 38–39
  Curried Cauliflower Soup, 76
  German Potato Salad, 40–41
  Ham and Potato Soup, 140–141
  Kielbasa and Vegetable
    Stew, 131
  Scalloped Potatoes with
    Smoked Salmon, 90–91
  Smashed Red Potatoes with
    Bacon, 48
  Spanish Tortilla, 31
  Vegetable Korma, 86–87
Pot-in-pot cooking, 4
Pressure cook/manual setting, 4, 15
Pressure release valves, 3
Proteins. *See also specific*
    portion guidelines, 10
Provolone cheese
  Italian Pork Sandwiches,
    136–137

Q
Quick release, 4
Quinoa
  Quinoa with Marinated
    Artichokes and Peppers, 71

R
Ramekins, 9
Recipe conversions, 18
Rice
  Artichoke and Spinach
    Risotto, 82
  Basic White or Brown Rice, 163
  Brown Rice and Broccoli
    Cheese Casserole, 61

Browned Butter Risotto, 42
Coconut-Vanilla Rice
    Pudding, 147
Congee with Eggs and
    Spinach, 25
Creamy Salsa Verde
    Chicken, 105
Herbed Wild Rice Pilaf with
    Almonds, 66
Jamaican Rice and Peas,
    68–69
Rice Pilaf with Bacon and
    Water Chestnuts, 64–65
Shawarma-Style Chicken and
    Rice, 106–107
Teriyaki Chicken and Rice, 113
Thai Red Curry Beef, 129–130
Ricotta cheese
  Mixed-Up Lasagna, 133
  Ricotta Cheesecakes
    with Balsamic
    Strawberries, 152–153
  Savory Ham and Cheese Egg
    Cups, 35
Rosemary
  Italian Pork Sandwiches,
    136–137
  Roasted Sweet Potatoes and
    Beets with Rosemary, 46

S
Salads
  Beet Salad with Creamy Dill
    Dressing, 44
  German Potato Salad, 40–41
  Greek Salad with Bulgur
    Wheat, 62
  Italian Tuna and Bean
    Salad, 102–103
  Southwestern Black Bean
    Salad, 60
  Tangy Carrot and Celery
    Salad, 45
  Warm Thai-Style Green Bean
    and Tomato Salad, 50–51
Salmon
  Farfalle with Salmon, Fennel,
    and Tomatoes, 92–93
  Scalloped Potatoes with
    Smoked Salmon, 90–91

Sandwiches
  Barbecue Chicken Sandwiches
    with Slaw, 116–117
  French Onion Soup Dip
    Sandwiches, 126–127
  Italian Pork
    Sandwiches, 136–137
Sauces
  Marinara Sauce, 160
Sausage
  Chicken Thighs with Salami
    and Fennel, 110–111
  Chorizo and Green Chile
    Breakfast Casserole,
    32–33
  Kielbasa and Vegetable
    Stew, 131
  Mixed-Up Lasagna, 133
  Penne with Italian Sausage and
    Broccoli Rabe, 132
  Pinto Beans with
    Chorizo, 58–59
Sauté setting, 4
Sealing rings, 3
Seals, 3
Shrimp
  Cilantro-Coconut Shrimp and
    Broccoli, 100
  Shrimp and Grits, 98–99
Soups and stews
  Beef Stew, 124–125
  Chicken Noodle Soup, 115
  Chicken Stock, 158
  Clam Chowder, 96–97
  Creamy Mushroom-Barley
    Soup, 70
  Curried Cauliflower Soup, 76
  Easy Chili, 123
  Ham and Potato Soup, 140–141
  Kielbasa and Vegetable
    Stew, 131
  Minestrone, 74–75
  Mushroom Stock, 159
  North African Chickpea
    Stew, 57
  White Bean Stew with Broccoli
    Rabe, 56
Spinach
  Artichoke and Spinach
    Risotto, 82

Congee with Eggs and
Spinach, 25
Minestrone, 74–75
Squash. *See also* Zucchini
Spaghetti Squash with Browned
Butter and Parmesan, 77
Steam setting, 4
Steamer baskets, 9
Sweet potatoes
Roasted Sweet Potatoes and
Beets with Rosemary, 46

T

Thyme
French Onion Soup Dip
Sandwiches, 126–127
Herbed Wild Rice Pilaf with
Almonds, 66
Jamaican Rice and Peas, 68–69
Roasted Sweet Potatoes and
Beets with Rosemary, 46
Tofu
Spicy Braised Tofu and
Carrots, 80
Tomatoes
Chicken Paprikash, 112
Chicken Thighs with Salami
and Fennel, 110–111
Easy Chili, 123
Farfalle with Salmon, Fennel,
and Tomatoes, 92–93
Greek Salad with Bulgur
Wheat, 62

Italian Tuna and Bean
Salad, 102–103
Marinara Sauce, 160
Minestrone, 74–75
North African Chickpea
Stew, 57
Penne with Italian Sausage and
Broccoli Rabe, 132
Pinto Beans with
Chorizo, 58–59
Polenta with Mushroom
Sauce, 78–79
Rotini with Creamy Basil and
Sun-Dried Tomato Sauce, 81
Thai Red Curry Beef, 129–130
Tomato, Mozzarella, and Basil
Quiche, 34
Vegetable Korma, 86–87
Warm Thai-Style Green Bean
and Tomato Salad, 50–51
Tortillas
Pork Tacos with Pineapple
Salsa, 138–139
Tuna
Italian Tuna and Bean
Salad, 102–103
Turkey
Turkey and Stuffing for
Two, 118–119

V

Vegetables. *See also specific*
portion guidelines, 11

Venting, 4
Vinegar, balsamic
Asparagus with Balsamic and
Pine Nuts, 49
Ricotta Cheesecakes with
Balsamic Strawberries,
152–153

W

Water chestnuts
Rice Pilaf with Bacon and
Water Chestnuts, 64–65
Spicy Chicken Lettuce
Cups, 108–109

Y

Yogurt
Small-Batch Yogurt, 164–165
Yogurt, Greek
Beet Salad with Creamy Dill
Dressing, 44
Ginger-Oatmeal Muffins, 23
North African Chickpea
Stew, 57
Shawarma-Style Chicken and
Rice, 106–107

Z

Zucchini
Minestrone, 74–75
Thai Red Curry Beef, 129–130

Acknowledgments

Special thanks to Stacy Wagner-Kinnear and Jenny Croghan at Callisto, who went above and beyond in their support for me and this book. Thanks also to Julie Kerr, who made the book better. Thanks to my assiduous recipe testers from eGForums at eGullet.org: Kerry Beal, Elise Bradley, Kay Brockwell, Elsie Mallon, Anna Nielsen, and Nancy (Smithy) Smith. And thanks to Caitlin. If it's true, as John Steinbeck said, "In writing, your audience is one single reader," then she was my audience for this book.